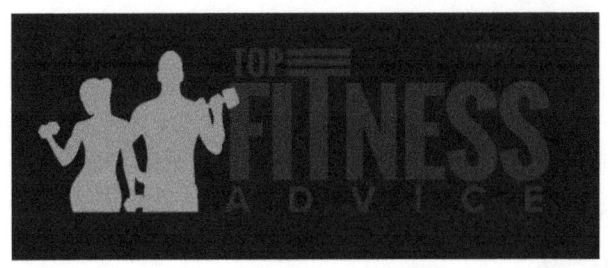

WEIGHT LOSS SMOOTHIES

4th Edition

9-Day Detox & Cleanse – Over 50 Smoothie Recipes Included

LINDA WESTWOOD

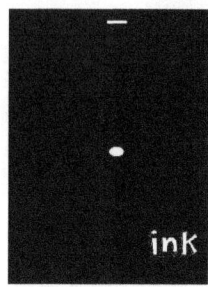

First published in 2015 by Venture Ink Publishing

Copyright © Top Fitness Advice 2019

All rights reserved.

No part of this book may be reproduced in any form without permission in writing from the author. No part of this publication may be reproduced or transmitted in any form or by any means, mechanic, electronic, photocopying, recording, by any storage or retrieval system, or transmitted by email without the permission in writing from the author and publisher.

Requests to the publisher for permission should be addressed to publishing@ventureink.co

For more information about the contents of this book or questions to the author, please contact Linda Westwood at linda@topfitnessadvice.com

Disclaimer

This book provides wellness management information in an informative and educational manner only, with information that is general in nature and that is not specific to you, the reader. The contents of this book are intended to assist you and other readers in your personal wellness efforts. Consult your physician regarding the applicability of any information provided in this book to you.

Nothing in this book should be construed as personal advice or diagnosis, and must not be used in this manner. The information provided about conditions is general in nature. This information does not cover all possible uses, actions, precautions, side-effects, or interactions of medicines, or medical procedures. The information in this book should not be considered as complete and does not cover all diseases, ailments, physical conditions, or their treatment.

You should consult with your physician before beginning any exercise, weight loss, or health care program. This book should not be used in place of a call or visit to a competent health-care professional. You should consult a health care professional before adopting any of the suggestions in this book or before drawing inferences from it.

Any decision regarding treatment and medication for your condition should be made with the advice and consultation of a qualified health care professional. If you have, or suspect you have, a health-care problem, then you should immediately contact a qualified health care professional for treatment.

No Warranties: The author and publisher don't guarantee or warrant the quality, accuracy, completeness, timeliness, appropriateness or suitability of the information in this book, or of any product or services referenced in this book.

The information in this book is provided on an "as is" basis and the author and publisher make no representations or warranties of any kind with respect to this information. This book may contain inaccuracies, typographical errors, or other errors.

Liability Disclaimer: The publisher, author, and other parties involved in the creation, production, provision of information, or delivery of this book specifically disclaim any responsibility, and shall not be held liable for any damages, claims, injuries, losses, liabilities, costs, or obligations including any direct, indirect, special, incidental, or consequences damages (collectively known as "Damages") whatsoever and howsoever caused, arising out of, or in connection with the use or misuse of the site and the information contained within it, whether such Damages arise in contract, tort, negligence, equity, statute law, or by way of other legal theory.

Table of Contents

Disclaimer	3
Who is this book for?	7
What will this book teach you?	9
Chapter One: What is the 9-Day Smoothie Cleanse?	11
Chapter Two: Do Smoothies Really Work?	17
Chapter Three: Starting Up	21
Chapter Four: Game Plan	27
Chapter Five: Speed Up Your Weight Loss	65
Chapter Six: Long-Term Weight Loss	79
Chapter Seven: Breakfast Smoothies	87
Chapter Eight: Lunch Smoothies	113
Chapter Nine: Dinner Smoothies	141
Chapter Ten: Mini-Smoothies	159
Conclusion	185
Final Words	187

Would you prefer to listen to my book, rather than read it?

Download the audiobook version for free!

If you go to the special link below and sign up to Audible as a new customer, you can get the audiobook version of my book completely free.

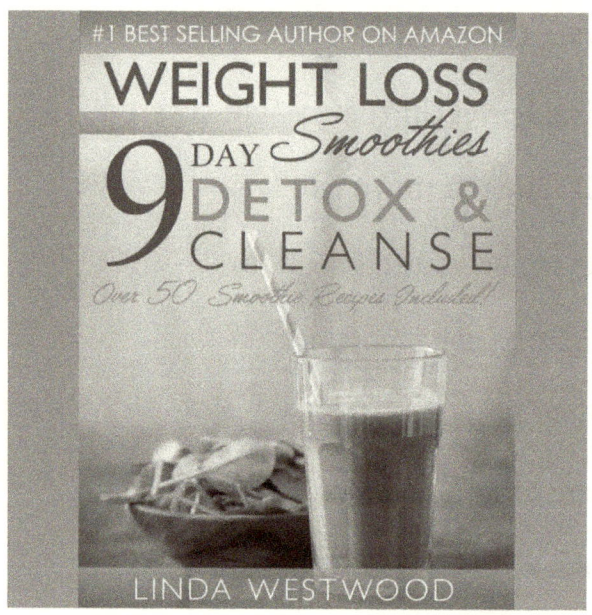

Go here to get your audiobook version for free:

TopFitnessAdvice.com/go/WeightSmoothies

Who is this book for?

Do you need a *strong* kick-start with your weight loss?

Are you constantly feeling tired and unhealthy throughout your day?

Do you just wish that your fat would just fall off *effortlessly?*

If you answered "Yes" to any of those questions – **this book is for you!**

I am going to share with you some of the best smoothies that will change your life!

I have put it all together in this awesome 9-Day Smoothie Cleanse plan that is set up for you to lose up to 17 pounds in just 9 days!

The best part about is that you don't even have to do any exercise!

You can be a complete beginner or someone who works out regularly, it doesn't matter!

If this sounds like it could help you, then keep reading...

What will this book teach you?

Inside, I will teach you one of the best 9-Day Smoothie Cleanses that will not only boost your weight loss, but also clear both your mind and body!

You will feel the healthiest you have ever felt – have the most energy you have ever had – and the fat will be melting *effortlessly!*

How?

Because you're going to consume a very healthy smoothie plan that specifically plans out when your body needs certain nutrients – and then gives them to you in those smoothie recipes.

In this book, I give you the plan right in front of you that will change your life – all you have to do is follow it!

One of the most important things for you to realize when reading this book is that this smoothie cleanse *really does work!*

However…

For you to achieve *real success*, you HAVE to apply this to your life.

This is where most people fail – they read through the entire book but do nothing.

You MUST try your best to apply as you read through the book!

Chapter One

What is the 9-Day Smoothie Cleanse?

This is going to be quite unlike any fast or cleanse that you have been on before. Conventional wisdom holds that you need to eat a lot of fruits and vegetables but says that all fats, protein and dairy need to be excluded.

Whilst this does seem to make sense, it is not actually all that accurate. Studies have indicated that the body can benefit from short periods of intermittent fasting. Fasting for two or three days, however, does not count as a short period.

If you are lactose intolerant, then you may benefit from cutting out dairy products, but there is no scientific reason to stop eating healthy fats and proteins. In fact, you may even be harming your health by doing so, especially if you fast for prolonged periods of time.

The 9-Day Smoothie Cleanse allows you to enjoy the best of both worlds. Your gastro-intestinal track gets a bit of a break because the food is already mashed up and your whole body benefits because of the flood of high quality nutrients you are getting.

In one way, the cleanse is the same as the more conventional fasts – junk foods, highly processed foods and refined foods are off the menu. You are also not allowed to consume anything that has refined sugar in it and cannot have coffee or normal tea.

It's not all doom and gloom for you java junkies though – you are allowed to drink green tea and this does have some caffeine in it. It may not give you as much caffeine as coffee but it can still give you a healthy buzz because it is loaded with antioxidants.

You are going to replace them with food that is bursting with flavor. The advantage here is that the plan is designed so that you get maximum detox benefits without needing to starve yourself or having to rely on unsatisfying vegetable broth to help you get through the day.

Protein and healthy fats are an essential part of any eating plan. If your body does not get enough protein from the food you eat, it starts to use the protein stored in your muscles.

Fat, unfortunately, has the opposite effect – if you are not getting enough, the body will minimize its usage of fat and try to store any fat that it is receiving.

From this standpoint, it is difficult to see why anyone fasts at all. It is too much of a drastic measure, especially when you can get much better results by just doing the smoothie cleanse.

The key is in using quality ingredients in your smoothie and by mixing up the recipes a bit. Even though you have to have at least one smoothie a day, it need not always be the same recipe.

The proponents of fasts make it sound as though your body is completely inefficient when it comes to getting rid of waste. The truth is somewhat different – your body is busy detoxing itself right now.

Because of our typical modern lifestyles, this process may not be as efficient as it should be – we pile toxins into our bodies all the time.

A good analogy is a tennis player paying against one of those machines that automatically lobs the ball. Initially, the player manages quite well because the balls are not lobbed as fast.

After a while though, the balls keep coming faster and faster and our tennis player is getting more and more tired. He will get to a point where he gets overwhelmed unless someone steps in to help him.

To continue this analogy, the plan acts as an assistant for the player – reducing the speed of the ball machine and also helping the player by catching balls that he missed.

This plan basically works with your body to make the detoxification process more efficient by reducing the toxic load on the body and by providing your internal organs with the support that they need to function at full speed.

It is this process that helps you to lose up to 15 pounds in 9 days.

Discover Scientifically-Proven "Shortcuts" & "Hacks" to Lose Weight FASTER (With Very Little Effort)

For this month only, you can get Linda's best-selling & most popular book absolutely free – *Weight Loss Secrets You NEED to Know.*

Get Your FREE Copy Here:
TopFitnessAdvice.com/Bonus

Discover scientifically-proven tips to help you lose weight faster and easier than ever before. With this book, readers were able to improve their weight loss results and fitness levels. So, it's highly recommended that you get this book, especially while it's free!

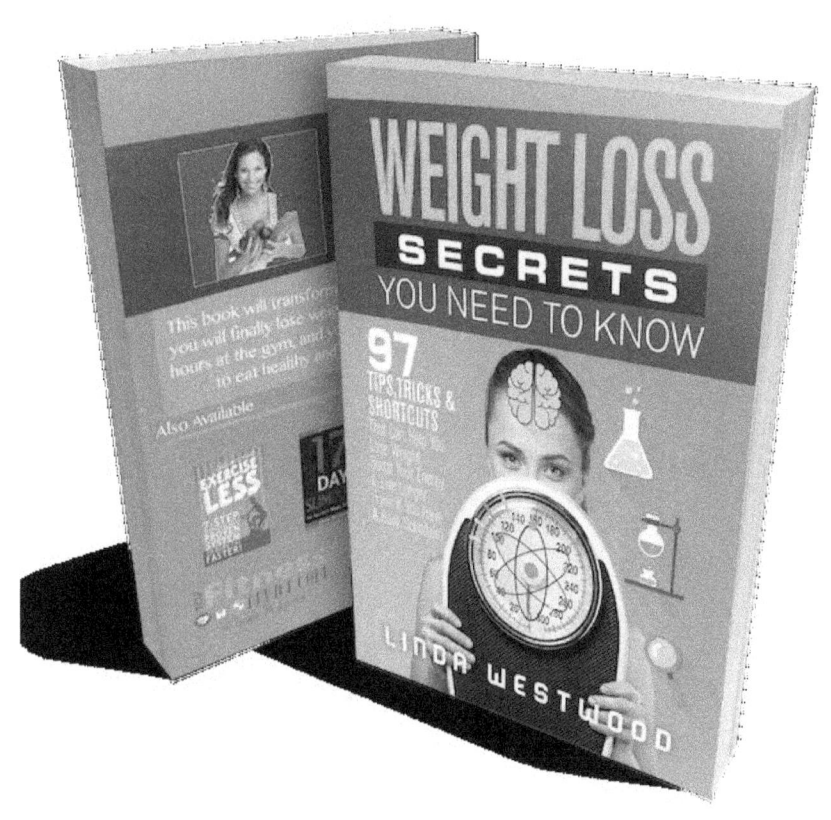

Get Your FREE Copy Here:

TopFitnessAdvice.com/Bonus

Chapter Two

Do Smoothies Really Work?

There has been a lot of press in the last few years about the benefits of drinking your nutrients in the form of smoothies and juices.

There are those that say that juicing is lot better and that it will help you to lose weight.

There are those who say that you have to eat "real" food and cannot "drink" your meals.

Others say that smoothies are too high in calories.

The truth lies in the middle ground – with smoothies, you are drinking your food but you are still getting all the fiber that you would have in the "real" food.

Most people actually start getting the right amounts of fiber for the first time in their lives because smoothies can be loaded with healthy foods and still taste good.

Smoothies do tend to have a lot of calories in them, but this is only if you make them incorrectly.

If, on the other hand, you follow the recipes in this book and you make them with the right ingredients, you will find that they are low-calorie recipes!

Remember that your body does need lots of calories a day to sustain it – the big problem with fad diets is that they reduce the caloric intake to such an extent that your body feels as though it is starving and holds onto any calories that it can.

That is one of the reasons why you often gain weight so soon after going on one of the fad diets.

Super Smoothie to the Rescue

This is where smoothies come in. You add a whole fruit or veggie into a smoothie – and this will maintain its already high fiber content!

The blending does break down some of the fiber content but, on the whole, you are still getting your daily dose of fiber and the impact on blood sugar levels is not nearly as great as in the case of, say, store-bought fruit juice. You will get enough of each type of fiber – soluble and insoluble.

Soluble fiber is absorbed into the blood stream and helps to mop up excess LDL cholesterol, keeping your heart healthier. Oats are a great source of soluble fiber and that is why you will see them in some of the recipes.

Insoluble fiber is just as important – it makes you feel fuller for longer and it is essential for the health of the good bacteria in our guts; it helps the food move as it should through the digestive tract and helps you stay regular.

Vegetables and fruits contain some insoluble fiber and some soluble fiber. Let's face it - nature wants us to eat fruit and veggies whole.

Smoothies offer a bit of a compromise – you get adequate fiber and a shot of vitamins and minerals in quantities that are closer to what nature originally intended, in a convenient liquid form.

Your average smoothie contains about the same amount of food that you should be eating in terms of a healthy, natural diet. The high levels of nutrients in the smoothies give your body what it needs to repair itself and so you will find that cravings go away.

The fresh ingredients in the smoothies are packed with antioxidants and so will help to fight the signs of aging and inflammation. They will also help to flush toxins out of your system.

Additionally, you won't really feel as hungry as you used to because smoothies are very filling. You can even tailor the types of smoothies that you drink so that you get the optimal benefits for your own personal condition – do you have a lot of problems with inflammation? Make sure you add plenty of nuts and seeds.

Need to get rid of gout? Celery is great at balancing the levels of uric acid in your system.

Smoothies taste good, are easy to prepare and fit in perfectly if you need to eat on the run. They are the perfect way to lose weight – you just need to put the right ingredients in.

I hope that you are enjoying this book so far, and if you could spare 30 seconds, I would greatly appreciate you leaving a review on Amazon.com.

Chapter Three

Starting Up

Getting Your Head Around the Concept

Being mentally prepared is the key to success. You are going to completely upend your diet and, initially at least, this is going to mean some adjustments.

Let's face it; you are going to be in for some discomfort – no change that is worthwhile is completely painless. That said, the discomfort is not going to be as extreme as it would be if you were fasting – you are still getting all the food groups that you need.

For those coffee junkies out there, this will be a little tough but that is why we have included green tea as well. You can drink up to 3 cups of green tea a day and, because of the caffeine content of the tea, caffeine withdrawal will not be as pronounced.

The tea should have no milk in it and should be sweetened with stevia or a little honey. It is because of the symptoms of detoxing that I advise starting over a weekend. By Monday or Tuesday morning you will be feeling a whole lot better – you just need to get through the first weekend.

The Epsom salts baths will also help to soothe the aches and pains and to speed up this initial detox period so that will help as well.

Any discomfort that you undergo is going to be short-lived anyway. Keep that in mind and you'll get through it.

Smoothies are Complete Meals

We are used to looking at smoothies as a nice side beverage. Consequently, we tend to look at a plan like this one and think that we are going to starve. What must be remembered is that smoothies are real meals.

With this plan, the smoothie recipes have been carefully chosen to provide a balanced meal.

You get enough fiber to help you feel full and the nutrients provided will give a smooth supply of energy without the spikes and crashes that make you feel ravenous.

Preparation of Food

Set aside some time to look out for good, healthy fruits and vegetables. Go to your local farmer's market nice and early in the morning to get the best selection of fruits, vegetables and herbs.

It is best to try and get locally grown, organic produce. Also look for products like raw milk, kefir, farm butter, etc. These usually taste a lot better than the store-bought varieties and are a lot less likely to be laced with chemicals and preservatives.

If there is an organic farm nearby, find out whether or not they deliver vegetable/fruit boxes – many of the organic farms offer to deliver to your home or office and they make up a box of the fruits and vegetables that were ripe and ready for harvest. Remember that organically grown produce may not look as perfect as the stuff that you find in the stores. The upside is that it probably hasn't been subjected to a lengthy storage process and long cold-food chain. The imperfections are a sign that the produce is natural and good for you.

Don't be afraid to try different combinations – as you will see in the recipe section, there are a lot of different options – white beans in a smoothie, for example, make it creamier.

Kefir provides a great source of protein and calcium but also provides valuable probiotics as well. Switching up the base fruit, the other fruits and the fats used is important because it gives you access to a much wider variety of nutrients.

Prepare as Much as Possible

If the morning is a mad rush for you, you might want to consider getting up 15 minutes earlier so that you have a bit more time.

You can, however, also cut back on the time needed to make your smoothies every morning as follows:

- *Keep all the necessary ingredients together* – set aside space in the kitchen cupboard to keep all of your smoothie spices, nuts and seeds together.

  You can even make little packs with the right amount of nuts, seeds and spices for one smoothie in each.

- *If you want to, you can chop up your fruit and vegetables the night before, put them in an airtight bag and freeze them.*

  This saves you having to put ice in the smoothie and saves time in the morning.

- *When you have to grind seeds, like with flaxseeds, it is best to do that just before you are ready to use them.*

  You can, however, measure out how much you need and get it ready in the grinder, or for those of us less technically inclined, in the mortar and pestle.

- Plan the day ahead and think about what smoothies you are going to make the night before you make them to ensure that you do have all the necessary ingredients before you start to prepare your smoothies.

What You Will Need

You need to start off with a good blender. It doesn't have to have every bell and whistle, but get the best quality that you can afford.

Here are some things that you should consider:

- **How powerful the motor is** – You want a bit more of a powerful motor here because you will be chopping nuts and ice. Look for motors that are 500 watts and up.

- **How easy it is to wash** – Ideally, you should be able

to disassemble the blade attachment and the actual jug of the blender from one another to be able to properly clean it out.

This is pretty important – if the blender is tough to clean, it could end up being more trouble than it is worth to use it.

- **The strength of the jar** – I have used blenders with plastic jars and those with glass jars. In my experience, the glass one stands up better over time.

- **How many speeds it has** – With blending, you need only three settings – Pulse, and two different blending speed buttons.

My blender has these settings – I usually only use the lowest speed. Occasionally, when a piece of fruit or vegetable is being stubborn, I use the pulse setting.

There are blenders out there that have several speed settings – this makes no difference, even my old, clapped out blender can blend a smoothie in less than a minute.

Tips for When You Are Making Your Smoothies

- Always put the fruits, veggies, nuts and fillers in first and ensure that there are no pieces bigger than a golf ball. This ensures a nice smooth result.

- Add in the liquids.

- Secure the lid and blitz for about half a minute.

- Check to see that everything got blended and make sure that there are no bits of fruit that got stuck under the blades.

- If you are adding any protein powders or spices, add them now.

- If you plan to add ice blocks, now is the time. Add them no more than two at a time, at most.

Check the manufacturer's manual ahead of time to ensure that your blender can handle ice. If you have added in frozen fruit, you can skip the ice. Consider adding frozen fruit or ice, especially when the weather is warm, it takes the smoothie up a notch if it is ice cold.

Check the consistency of the smoothie – if it is too thick, add more ice or water; if it is too thin, you can add more fruit or filler.

Chapter Four

Game Plan

How to Use this Book

The smoothie recipes in this book have been broken up into Breakfast, Lunch, Dinner and Mini-Smoothies, each with their own chapter. Every day, replace your Breakfast, Lunch and Dinner with a smoothie from the appropriate section.

If you find that you are feeling hungry between meals, choose a mini-smoothie and have that.

In the mini-smoothie section I have also included smoothies that are good for specific health complaints like colds and flu, gout, etc. All mini-smoothies can be converted, in need, to full smoothies – just check what you need to add in terms of the guidelines and go from there.

If you do convert it, it needs to count as a full meal. The rules for this cleanse are simple – you must have three full smoothies a day, one of which must be a green one; you may have one mini-smoothie between meals if you are really hungry; you need to drink a minimum of 8 glasses of water and three cups of plain green tea a day (if you miss your coffee).

I recommend that you have your green smoothie for breakfast but you could switch it for lunch if you wanted to. Most of the smoothies can be switched to different times of day.

One word of caution though, be careful when it comes to switching out the evening ones – the breakfast and lunch smoothies have been designed to provide more energy than the dinner ones have.

If you decide to have a breakfast smoothie for dinner, make sure to have it at least 4-5 hours before bedtime. Don't just dismiss a smoothie out of hand because of one ingredient – unless you have a specific allergy to it – try the smoothie first. You'll be amazed at how different things taste when they've been whizzed together.

Naturally, not every item in every smoothie will appeal to everyone. If that is the case, you can do some substitutions when it comes to ingredients, based on the principles that I share with you below.

You can also feel free to add extra herbs or spices to the existing recipes if that interests you. Do not, however, add extra nuts or seeds as these are very calorie dense. Once you start getting the hang of how to put together a smoothie, you'll have fun experimenting.

The Basics a Smoothie Should Have for Weight Loss

There are tons of recipes available but basically, they all come down to a few ingredients.

Here is what every smoothie should have in it:

- The base – this is going to be something like water, milk, or non-dairy milks
- A serving of fruit for flavor
- A source of high-quality protein
- Some veggies
- A source of healthy fat
- Some sort of filler – to make the smoothie more filling. Oats is an easy one to use.
- Optional extras like sweeteners, etc.

The Base

The base is what will bind the other smoothie ingredients together and what makes it more drinkable. Some people use a base of plain water; others use milk, yoghurt or dairy alternatives.

Coconut water and milk are just some of the alternatives that you can consider. Experiment with different bases to see which ones you enjoy best and which ones work best for you.

The best news? Low-fat is now being shown to be bad for you so use the full-fat versions instead. As long as there is no added sugar in the milk you are using, it is good for you.

Almond Milk

Make Your Own Almond Milk

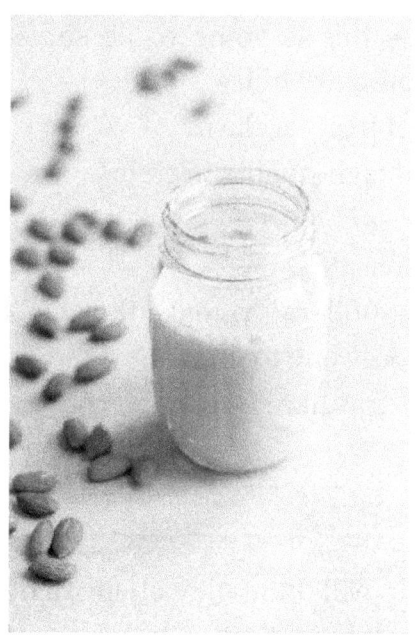

It is always better to make just enough to keep you going for a couple of days.

You will need:

- A blender
- Something to strain the milk with
- A container to keep the milk in – preferably airtight
- 500g almonds
- 3 cups of water for every cup of almonds used
- 5ml vanilla essence

Soak the almonds overnight in the water. In the morning, whizz them up in the blender. Strain out the almond meal and put to one side. Mix in the vanilla essence and your milk is ready.

I add about a third of the almond milk back into the smoothie and keep the rest in a covered container in the refrigerator.

You will use about a cup or two of the milk per smoothie, depending on what other ingredients you are using as well and also depending on how thick you want the end result to be.

You can also use the milk as a healthy dairy alternative. Use as is or reduce the amount of water added in order to get a creamier result.

Bonus Tip: The almond milk makes a nourishing, cleansing skin mask. Apply to skin while still damp and massage a little. Leave on for about 10-15 minutes before rinsing off. Almond oil has long been used in cosmetics to nourish dry skin. The almond milk also exfoliates the skin, leaving it smoother and soothed.

What About Milk?

You can always, if you want to, use milk or yoghurt instead of almond milk. The almond milk has got more nutrients and will give you more energy but it is not always a practical idea.

If you are rushing, you can use normal milk or yoghurt to thicken the smoothie.

The milk, yoghurt or almond milk makes up the base and also the protein content for the smoothie. This will help to slow the absorption of glucose into the blood stream so do not skip this step.

If you are going to use milk, add in the same quantities that you would for almond milk. If you are using yoghurt, the end result will be creamier and thicker so be sure to compensate by adding extra water.

Do use natural, unsweetened yoghurt and steer clear of any flavored yoghurt – the trick with the smoothies is to make them as healthy as possible and this means avoiding added sugar.

Another alternative is to use a milk product called Kefir. Buy Kefir made from cow's milk NOT goat's milk.

The one from cow's milk is a lot subtler and you will not taste it in your smoothie. The goat's milk one tastes and smells awful, I don't care how good it is for you (my opinion).

If you have access to raw milk, you can use a little left over Kefir to start your own batch. You just sterilize a jar and let it cool, add about 2 cups of milk and about ½ a cup of kefir.

Put it in a cool dark place for about three days until it resembles what you'd originally bought and then store it in the fridge. (It will stay okay for about a week or so once in the fridge).

Coconut Water or Milk?

It may sound odd to speak of adding coconut water or milk to a healthy smoothie – we have all been led to believe that coconut milk has a high fat content. That is very true but it is also true that it is a high-quality fat that our bodies can put to great use.

Coconut water has high levels of electrolytes and essential nutrients. Coconut milk is extremely nourishing and tasty.

Make Your Own Coconut Milk

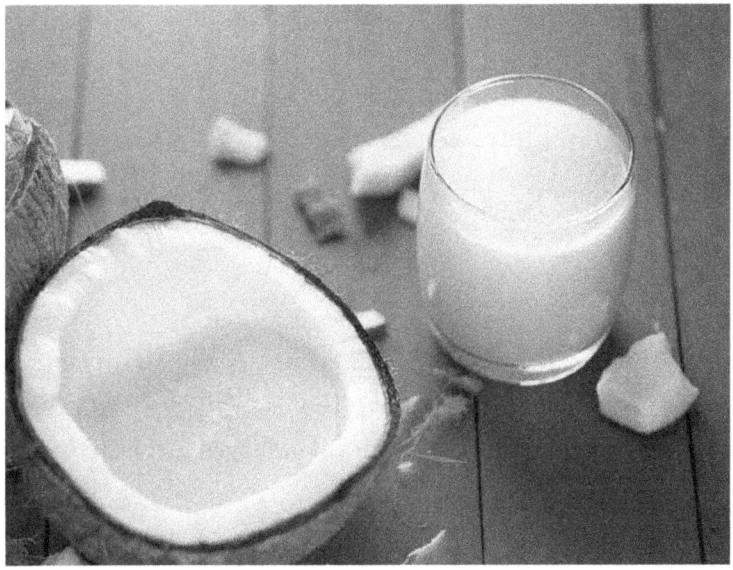

As with almond milk, make enough to last at most three days.

Ingredients

- 1 cup dried coconut – no sugar please
- 3 cups boiling water
- Pinch of salt
- Cheesecloth or tea towel to catch the bits
- Strainer

Method

1. Place the coconut into the water and leave it to soak for at least 10-15 minutes.

2. Blend until as smooth as possible and then place in the tea towel/cheesecloth into the strainer over a bowl.

3. Let as much of the liquid drain through as possible and then squeeze out the rest.

4. Keep the bit left over to either add to smoothies as extra filling or use when baking.

Fruit is Served

Adding fruit into the smoothie is about more than just adding nutrients, it is also about adding flavor. The fruit adds a touch of sweetness that makes the smoothie taste a whole lot better. (This allows you to sneak in those other veggies that you are not that keen on).

What you do want to be careful of is adding too much fruit because it has a lot of sugar in it. You need to be careful about the G.I. of the fruit that you decide to add – you may add one serving of fruit with a high G.I. and one with a lower G.I.

Generally speaking, the sweeter the fruit, the higher the sugar content is. You can add whatever fruit you like – it is pretty much all good for you, as long as you watch the serving size. Try to stick to fruit that is in season – it not only tastes better but tends to be fresher and more nutritious as well.

If you are really battling to find good fresh fruit, frozen will also be okay. Dried fruit is out completely – it has a lot of fiber but too much sugar that goes with it. Fruit in the blender is easy – if you can eat the skin of the fruit, simply wash well, chop into quarters, remove the stone, if applicable, and throw into the blender.

You don't need to peel or core the piece of fruit. In fact, adding in the skin is much better for you anyway. I also don't worry too much about coring the fruit or getting rid of the pips inside. They really don't make that much of a difference anyway so you don't need to waste your time removing pips.

Do, however, remove fruit stones as these can damage your blender. For this plan, you may add two servings of fruit at most. Switch out the fruits that you use so that you get a variety of fruits and thus a variety of minerals.

If you want more variety, nothing is stopping you from adding 4 different half servings of fruit.

Freeze!

During summer, it is great to have a cold smoothie in the morning. Using frozen fruit can help make the smoothie taste good without you having to worry about diluting the flavor with ice.

If you are pressed for time in the morning, prepare your fruit the night before and freeze it so that it is ready the next morning.

Suitable Fruits for Smoothies

- ***Berries*** – fresh and frozen. It's a good idea to always have at least one tub of berries on standby in your freezer.

    That way, if you are rushed in the morning or were unable to get fresh fruit, you still have options.

    Berries are high in fiber and lower in natural sugars so they are a healthier option when it comes to blood sugar control. You could, for example, eat a whole tub of strawberries (no sugar added) without worrying unduly about spiking your blood sugar.

    Blueberries are best in terms of anti-oxidant power so do have them at least once or twice a week if you are able to.

- ***Bananas*** – One of the stalwarts for a number of smoothie recipes, bananas are a great addition because of their sweet flavor and creamy texture.

    They contain a lot of magnesium and can help you to sleep because of this. They also help fill you up. You should not, however, put more than one banana in because they are so full of sugar.

    Bananas freeze rather well – do blend them while frozen though because they become very mushy when defrosted.

- ***Pears and Apples*** – Both fruits are great for making smoothies with. They add flavor, fiber and nutrients without adding too much sugar.

- ***Pineapples*** – Pineapples are the only dietary source of Bromelain, an enzyme that is known to aid the digestion, help alleviate inflammation and pain and assist in the treatment of arthritis and rheumatism.

  If you have an upset stomach, add pineapple to your smoothie – it will help.

- ***Grapefruit and Lemons*** – Grapefruit and lemons are great for weight loss. Try to use a non-dairy base if using these two fruits as the juice may curdle milk or yoghurt.

  Grapefruits have been proven to be an effective weight loss tool – they stimulate the fat burning mechanisms within the body.

- ***Coconut*** – Coconut milk can provide a very creamy flavor to the smoothies and will help you to feel fuller. Alternatively, add pieces of fresh coconut, desiccated coconut or even coconut oil.

  Coconut can boost the action of the liver and so is helpful in detoxification. In addition, the fruit is very high in nutrients and fiber.

- ***Pomegranates*** – These are one of nature's super foods. They are rich in nutrients and have been shown to have appetite-suppressing effects. They have also proven useful in reducing the levels of LDL cholesterol in the blood and in helping the body detoxify.

- **Mangoes** – Mangoes are great in smoothies. Do restrict your intake to one a day though as they are high in natural sugars. That said, they are very high in Vitamin C and help create a creamier, sweeter smoothie.

  Smoothies are ideal for mangoes – eating the fruit as is can be very messy and can cause sores to form around the mouth. Adding them to a smoothie solves both of these problems.

- **Papayas** – Papayas also have their share of natural sugars but are not as bad as bananas and mangoes. They also stimulate the digestive enzymes and thus help the digestive tract along.

  These fruits are also high in Vitamin C and taste great. Do make sure though that the papaya is properly ripe before eating it – if it is green it can cause a running stomach.

- **Passion Fruit** – The pulp inside is full of flavor and full of Vitamin C. These make great addition to both the taste and appearance of the smoothie. If you cannot find the fresh fruit, you can, in this instance use canned, as long as there is no added sugar or preservatives.

Bonus Tip: When it comes to the peels that you cannot eat, don't just throw them out. You can make yourself a quick beauty treatment.

Wash your face and then rub the inside of the banana or papaya peel all over. Leave for a few minutes before rinsing off and you'll have given your skin a boost.

A Source of High-Quality Protein

Protein is essential in this plan – it helps you to feel fuller for longer, helps in the building of lean muscle mass and revs up the metabolism. You should eat a serving of protein with every meal. Your base will provide some protein content, but you need more than that.

Whilst it is tempting to turn to a protein powder, this is not the best idea if you want to lose weight. Rather stick to natural sources of protein such as nuts, seeds and yoghurt.

Alternatively, you can look to adding in more nuts or seeds to increase the protein content significantly. Chia seeds, for example, have very high protein content.

Tofu also provides a nutritious alternative to more traditional protein sources, especially if you are lactose intolerant or are allergic to nuts.

Get Your 5 Veggies A Day

The biggest benefit when it comes to smoothies though is that you can throw in just about anything when it comes to vegetables. Because the ingredients are blended up, the taste is masked. This is great for those who are not fans of vegetables. You can choose any vegetable as long as it can be eaten raw. Choose the freshest vegetables that you can find – if possible, grow your own.

All you want to have to do by way of preparing the vegetables is to scrub them clean and add them to the smoothie. With vegetables especially, most of the fiber is in the skins so if you peel them you will be missing out.

Do try to vary the types of vegetables that you use from day to day and try to get a good mix between different types of vegetables for maximum nutritional benefit.

If you really want to, you can steam the vegetables lightly before adding them. It is really best to eat them raw though.

Sprouts

When it comes to life giving nutrients, there is little that can compare to sprouted seeds. It is well worth considering sprouting your own seeds as an additive to your smoothies, especially when you are eating green smoothies.

Sprouting is easy – all you need to do is to soak the seeds overnight, drain the water off and place them in a glass jar. Place a piece of muslin over the opening of the jar and leave the sprouts in a dark, cool place.

Rinse with water every morning and evening. In a few days' time, they'll be ready to eat. You want to eat them when the roots and stalks are about 1cm long. Once you have harvested them you can store them in an air-tight container in the refrigerator. Stored in this manner they have a shelf-life of about a week.

Be meticulous about rinsing the sprouts properly – if you don't, they can attract mold and fungus. If you detect a sour smell or there seems to be fungal growth, discard the sprouts. With practice though, that will seldom happen.

Once you really get the hang of it, you'll never be without sprouts again. To make it even easier, you can use sprouting trays in place of the bottle.

Also, always be sure to buy seeds meant for sprouting. Seeds packed for planting are not suitable as they are usually chemically treated.

The Benefits of Sprouts

- Sprouts have hardly any calories and lots of fiber. They bulk out your smoothie without adding significant amounts of calories. Sprouts can be very filling foods.

- Their flavor is quite different from that of the vegetable that they will grow into – it's a lot sweeter and a bit milder.

- They are a good source of nutrients and protein.

- They are alkalizing in the body – they help to reduce high levels of acid and thus contribute to the fight against inflammation.

- Eating them on a regular basis makes will help maintain your proper sodium balance and so also help to control problems with blood pressure.

- Sprouts contain digestive enzymes and also help to balance the blood sugar levels within our bodies.

- They increase detoxification by significant levels.

What Sprouts to Use

- ***Alfalfa*** – Alfalfa is one of the most nutritious sprouts that you can grow. It is not by accident that it is so popular as cattle fodder and green compost.

    It has high protein content and is packed with vitamins and minerals. Added to your daily smoothie it will assist in detoxification, act as a tonic for the immune system and provide a seeming limitless supply of energy.

    If you are only going to choose one plant to sprout, it should be alfalfa. The roots of the alfalfa plant go deep into the soil – much deeper than in other plants and this allows it access to more nutrients than most plants.

    The sprouts have a slightly sweet taste.

- ***Barley*** – Barley is extremely nutritious. Barley water has been used for centuries to treat a variety of conditions from stomach ailments to diabetes.

    Sprouts added to your smoothie will help to soothe inflammation and irritation and alkalinize the blood. Barley is also good for reducing the symptoms of hay fever.

- ***Fenugreek*** – Fenugreek seeds are easy to sprout and have a more peppery flavor. Added to your smoothie, Fenugreek will help to soothe digestive upsets, balance blood sugar and cholesterol levels.

    It is also a great additive for detoxifying and will help to boost immunity. It has a bit of a peppery flavor.

- ***Wheat grass*** - is high in nutrients and a great aid in detoxification. It will help give you energy, rev up the metabolism and will provide valuable anti-oxidants. It is particularly easy to grow at home and sprouting wheat grass is particularly rewarding. Wheat grass is sometimes sweet and sometimes a little bitter. I don't think that I would eat it on its own though.

    These are very rewarding plants to sprout – they grow incredibly quickly.

- ***Sunflower Seeds*** – When it comes to plant proteins, sunflower greens take a lot to beat. They have the complete range of amino acids that the body requires.

They provide support to the enzymes of the body and have amazing immune-boosting effects. These might not always sprout – it depends a lot on how old the seeds are – so don't be disappointed if they don't sprout.

- **Mustard and Radish Seeds** – These sprouts really easily and add a bit of a peppery flavor. Also packed with nutrients, both of these greens will help to boost the immune system and help to detoxify the system.

If you feel you have a bit of a cold coming on, mustard sprouts will clear it up in no time.

Other Vegetables to Include

When it comes to vegetables for your smoothies, the only "rule", as such, is to use the vegetables raw. That rules out vegetables such as potatoes and squashes but not too many others.

Wherever possible, leave the peel on – that is where a lot of the nutrients and fiber are. Scrub the vegetables well in need and simply chop them up roughly for inclusion in your smoothies.

If you are unsure about what vegetables to add, stick to vegetable staples like carrots, kale, etc. until you get the hang of things.

If you grow your own vegetables, or have a source at a farmer's market, you can get vegetables that haven't been topped or tailed. This is great – you can add the greens into your smoothie as well for an extra boost.

Do use vegetables that are in season and as fresh as possible. The beauty of the green smoothie is that it includes a wide range of things – the tops of carrots and beetroots, for example, can be just as healthy as the veggies themselves.

We usually throw them out because they don't taste as great. Blended into a smoothie, we barely taste them at all.

- **Kale** – Kale is similar in nutritional content to spinach but does not have the same high level of oxalates, making it the healthier choice for green smoothies.

  The problem with oxalates is that they, if taken regularly, cause kidney stones. Cooking helps to rid the spinach of some of these oxalates. For better health, raw kale is the better bet.

- **Carrots** –Carrots are a wonderful vegetable – full of fiber, sweet tasting and chock-full of anti-oxidants.

  Carrots make a great addition to any smoothie. Try using baby carrots for the ultimate in flavor and remember that you can also use the carrot greens in your smoothie as well.

- **Sea Vegetables** – Adding seaweed, etc. is a great way to source nutrients that we simply do not find in land vegetables.

The sulfated polysaccharides found in sea vegetables have anti-cancer, anti-thrombotic, anti-coagulant, anti-viral and anti-inflammatory properties.

You will also find them rich in various minerals such as zinc and copper, in quantities that are not present in land vegetables.

- ***Cucumber*** – Cucumber is a nice filler and has cooling properties. It does also have a range of nutrients but the skin is where the highest concentrations are.

  The skin is high in silica and Vitamin E. Cucumbers will also contribute to your daily Vitamin C quota.

- ***Beans, Peas and Legumes*** – Raw green beans and peas are great additions to your smoothie. They provide loads of fiber and nutrients.

  You can also use chick-peas, beans or lentils, as long as they have been sprouted. If you just throw in plain lentils or dried beans, your body will not be able to digest them properly and they will cause stomach upsets.

  To remember what can be added into this category, it is easiest to think about how you would prepare the legumes normally – if they need to be soaked before cooking them, they need to be sprouted before you can add them to the smoothie.

- ***Lettuce*** – Lettuce is not known as being a powerhouse of nutrients but it can help with the detox process. Where it is truly valuable, however, is in your dinner smoothie. It can help relax you and facilitate sleep.

Hey There Herb!

To really increase the potency of your smoothies, you are going to be adding in some herbs as well. It is really better, as far as possible, to add in fresh herbs, but dry herbs will do at a push. You will typically add in about 1/3 cup of fresh herbs or about a teaspoon of the dried herbs.

Don't ever use more than a teaspoon of the seeds at any one time and always ensure that the seeds are crushed just before adding to the smoothie.

As is the case with vegetable seeds, only use seeds that are specifically meant to be used for culinary purposes. Seeds meant for planting are usually chemically treated and not safe for consumption.

Do remember that herbs, whilst all natural, can be quite potent. It is not advisable to add more than the quantities quoted above unless you are under the supervision of a qualified naturopath.

Herbs are really easy to grow and don't take up too much space so there really is not reason why you shouldn't at least try to grow your own.

If push comes to shove, you can grow herbs in a pot on a sunny windowsill.

Benefits of Herbs in Smoothies

Herbs have all sorts of benefits and it will really depend on the actual herb that you use. Typically, they all contain nutrients and assist in detoxification. Herbs can be great for flavor as well.

I am going to list some of the more common herbs used in smoothies to aid weight loss but do keep in mind that this is not an exhaustive list. Do yourself a favor and read up more on the subject – it is well worth looking into.

- **Basil** – You can use Sweet Basil if you like for a nicer flavor. If you are looking for perennial basil, Sacred Basil is a good bet. (It does grow into a fairly big bush though so be warned.)

    Basil has a myriad of benefits but primary amongst these is the ability to detoxify the system. Basil has anti-bacterial properties and is an excellent anti-stress remedy.

- **Celery** – Celery is a super herb when it comes to detoxification. It has strong diuretic properties.

    It helps clean infections out of the bladder and kidneys and helps to clear out uric acid in the tissues. (This helps to relieve symptoms of gout, rheumatism, arthritis, etc.). It acts as an anti-spasmodic, lowers blood pressure and is generally a good tonic for the system.

Warning: If you are pregnant or suffer from any renal complaints, you should avoid using celery on a regular basis.

- **Cilantro** – Cilantro helps with digestion and boosts immunity. It also has a whole range of vitamins and minerals in it.

- **Cumin** – Fresh cumin leaves or flowers added to your smoothie will help with the detoxification process.

If you are finding that you are uncomfortable during this process due to flatulence, a teaspoon of crushed cumin seeds in your smoothie will provide some relief. You need to either crush or chew cumin seeds to get the full benefits.

- **Dandelion** – If you have been putting your system under a lot of pressure due to over-indulgence, dandelion is a good option. It cleanses and supports the liver.

It has diuretic properties but, unlike similar herbs, also as high levels of Potassium to replace that which is lost during the process. It also has diuretic properties.

- **Fennel** – Fennel has a licorice flavor that is quite pleasing. You can add it to both smoothies for the first three days to really jumpstart the detoxification process.

It is a great additive if you have been overdoing the food and alcohol. Do give yourself a break of at least 3 days after using for three days though. Either use 1/3 cup of the fresh leaves and flowers or a teaspoon of crushed seeds. Be prepared, it is a strong diuretic.

- **Mint** – The primary benefit of mint is as a digestive aid. Mint will ease an upset stomach and also help you to feel more alert. It can also help in the first few days to alleviate the headaches commonly associated with detox.

- **Parsley** – Parsley's primary benefit is as a diuretic and detoxifier. It is also packed with vitamins and is useful in the treatment of gout, flatulence, feverishness and high blood pressure.

- **Stevia** – Stevia is the ideal herb for those with a sweet tooth. It is extremely sweet and can replace sugar. Depending on where the Stevia is from, a couple of leaves can replace about a cup of sugar.

    It is great for weight loss as it sweetens and satisfies cravings for sugar. It has a positive impact on blood sugar levels, blood cholesterol levels and blood pressure. It also helps fight tooth decay.

It is best to add only one or two herbs to your smoothie overall or you could risk overpowering the flavor that you have created. Do experiment with different flavors – the right herb can lift the flavor beautifully.

Fat can help you lose weight!

Contrary to what we have been taught about fat, not all fat is bad for us. Your body needs fats to survive. The trick is to eat the right kinds of fats – fats the body can use. Nuts and seeds contain monounsaturated fats and these have been linked to increased insulin sensitivity, better health and loss of body fat.

Fats added to your smoothie will give you essential nutrients and will help you to feel fuller. They also add a satisfying creamy texture to the smoothie and help you to feel full for longer.

Here are some fats you can add:

- ***Nuts and Seeds*** - We have already spoken about the benefits of almonds and some of the benefits of sunflower greens but here we are going to look at other nuts and seeds as well.

    Nuts and seeds contain these fats and are packed with nutrients – vitamins, essential minerals, fiber and protein.

    The problem is that most people can't just stop at a single serving and that is when the trouble starts. Adding nuts and seeds to your smoothie instead helps you overcome this issue, allowing you to get the benefits without overindulging. You don't need to add a lot either, about a handful is enough.

- **Coconut Oil** - The fat in coconuts has actually been proven to shift the body's fat-burning mechanisms up a notch or two.

It is for this reason that people sometimes add coconut oil to their smoothies. (If adding oil, you need only add 1 tablespoon per smoothie to derive the benefits.) It also increases the satiety rating of whatever you eat meaning you can get away with eating less.

Coconut oil is considered the healthiest of all the fats.

- **Avocados** – These are one of nature's wonder foods and everyone should be eating them. Delicious, packed with nutrients, monounsaturated fats and fiber, avocados make great additions to green smoothies.

If you are only using half, leave the stone in the other half and place in the refrigerator. The stone keeps the other half from going brown.

- **Cream and Butter** – A tablespoon or two of either cream or butter adds a great taste and is super healthy – especially if the animals have been grass-fed.

Nuts to Add to Smoothies

- **Walnuts** - Fight inflammation. Walnuts have more antioxidants than any other nuts and so are great at fighting of the free radicals that damages the cells in our body. They also have the highest level of Omega-3 fatty acids and have particularly high levels of Manganese.

They reduce inflammation in the body overall and this, in turn, can help in the fight against painful conditions such as arthritis. Reduced inflammation also means a reduced chance of developing the so-called lifestyle diseases such as Heart Disease and Diabetes.

- *Almonds* – Almonds have more fiber and Vitamin E than any other nuts. A study published in the International Journal of Obesity found that the group who included almonds in their daily diet lost more weight overall than the group who didn't.

  Almonds offer powerful benefits in terms of protection against developing Diabetes. One study found that eating almonds daily decreased LDL Cholesterol levels and insulin resistance and consequently decreased the chances of disease.

  Almonds may also be good for the beneficial bacteria in your body. It is best if you can soak the almonds before use – overnight is ideal, if time permits.

- *Cashews* – Cashews shine when it comes to iron and zinc content. Iron is important in the fight against anemia and zinc is essential when it comes to your body's immunity against disease.

Cashews also provide significant amounts of magnesium – an essential mineral that most of us are deficient in. Magnesium can help protect you against dementia and Alzheimer's and is necessary for good brain health.

- **Pecans** – Pecans are also rich in antioxidants and have been shown to not only reduce the level of LDL Cholesterol but also to help prevent plaque forming in the arteries. The high Vitamin E content could also form a protective function in the brain, reducing the chances of developing diseases such as Lou Gehrig's or slowing their progression.

- **Brazil Nuts** – When it comes to Selenium, Brazil nuts are super stars. You can get your total recommended daily allowance from just one nut. Selenium may help to protect you against developing some types of cancer. In some studies, selenium has been shown to slow the growth of cancer cells.

  That said, you should not overdo it – getting too much Selenium can prove toxic to the body. Stick to one serving of Brazil nuts every other day to be on the safe side.

- **Macadamia Nuts** – Macadamias have a bad reputation for being fattening. They do have the most calories of all nuts but they also contain the highest levels of monounsaturated fats.

These fats help to reduce LDL cholesterol levels and can help in the fight against high blood pressure. Mix into a smoothie that contains cocoa for a pretty close to perfect chocolate taste.

- **Pistachios** – Pistachios are one of the least calorie dense nut so if you are worried about the calorie content, they are ideal. Pistachios have high levels of Gamma-Tocopherol – a type of Vitamin E especially useful in fighting cancer.

They also have a lot of potassium – vital for your central nervous system and the good heath of your musculature system. The B6 helps to improve mood and boosts immunity.

- **Hazelnuts** – Hazelnuts are rich in monounsaturated fats and Vitamin E making them heart healthy and very good for the skin. Hazelnuts can help prevent deterioration of the eyes, and the development of dementia.

Seeds to Add to Smoothies

- **Chia Seeds** – These are said to be one of the Aztecs biggest secrets. They were especially prized for providing energy, improving stamina and for their able to make the eater feel satiated. Soak them in water overnight before adding to your smoothie and they become more like porridge than seeds.

They are high in calcium, folate, iron, magnesium, soluble fiber and omega-3 fatty acids. They help to balance blood sugar and reduce inflammation in the body.

- **Hemp Seeds** – Hemp seeds do not have the same active ingredient found in marijuana so you cannot get high from eating them. They do, however, contain high levels of complete proteins and Omega-3 fatty acids.

- **Pumpkin Seeds** – These are rich in iron, B vitamins, magnesium, protein and zinc, as well as essential fatty acids.

Most important for the dieter, however, is the high levels of tryptophan – the amino acid that is the precursor of serotonin. This helps to reduce anxiety overall and will help you feel better able to cope.

- **Sunflower Seeds** – Ever wonder why your parrot is so chirpy? It's because he eats plenty of sunflower seeds. Sunflower seeds are full of B vitamins, Vitamin E, protein and Omega-3's.

- **Flax Seeds** – These seeds made a name for themselves as the best plant source of omega-3 fatty acids. There is so much more to them than that though. They also have a lot of soluble fiber – great for helping you feel full and for reducing blood cholesterol levels.

They also contain lots of lignans – a substance thought to protect against some types of cancer.

Spice it Up

Adding spices to your smoothies will not only make them taste better but will also allow you to enjoy greater health benefits as well. Spices are added in smaller quantities – a little goes a long, long way.

You can experiment with the different spices you have at home but there are a few spices that you need to try in at least one or two of your smoothies.

Spices to Use in Your Smoothies

- *Cinnamon* - Cinnamon is a powerful antioxidant, fights inflammation and has been scientifically proven to reduce levels of triglycerides and cholesterol. That's impressive but not as impressive as its effects in terms of the regulation of blood sugar.

    Cinnamon has been proven to reduce fasting blood sugar in diabetics by anywhere from 10% to 29%. That's a lot! All you need is to add ½ teaspoon to each smoothie daily.

- *Turmeric* – Turmeric has been proven to be an effective anti-inflammatory agent throughout the body. It is used in traditional Ayurvedic medicine to treat upset stomachs and acid reflux.

For the best effects, Turmeric should be taken with a meal that has some fat in it. (Making it perfect for your smoothies.) It is also best to take a few peppercorns at the same time to enhance the absorption of the curcumin – the active ingredient in turmeric.

In addition, curcumin is a potent anti-oxidant and can help to slow down the aging process and also protect against lifestyle diseases and age-related diseases such as Alzheimer's and Dementia.

It is also showing promise in the reversal of the damage done by heart disease and in the fight against depression. You would add 2 tablespoons of Turmeric to your smoothie.

- *Cayenne Pepper* – Cayenne Pepper is a dieter's friend – the capsaicin content helps to boost fat-burning and to curb appetite. You need to add about ¼ teaspoon to your smoothie to benefit.

    Cayenne Pepper revs up the metabolism and helps to speed up the lymphatic system. Blood circulation is boosted and it helps to regulate blood pressure.

    It is anti-bacterial, anti-fungal, anti-viral and anti-inflammatory. You can substitute cayenne pepper for paprika in need.

- *Ginger* – Ginger is also great at soothing digestive upsets and at promoting the detoxification process. It has strong anti-inflammatory properties and may help reduce pain in the body.

- ***Nutmeg*** – Nutmeg imparts a nice flavor and has excellent anti-inflammatory properties. It is also said to be a potent aphrodisiac!

Fillers

If there is enough fiber in a smoothie, it is pretty filling. Sometimes though, it is good to add a bit extra filling to help make you fuller. Choosing a healthy filler will further improve the benefits of the smoothie as a whole.

Here are some examples of fillers that you could add:

- ***Oatmeal*** – one of my favorites and I always use it raw. They help to balance high blood pressure, blood sugar levels, high cholesterol, and boost the immune system.

    They are packed with Vitamin B – vital for a healthy nervous system. They thus help beat stress. ½ to 1 cup of oats per smoothie will set you up with energy for the day ahead.

- ***Oat Bran*** – this is the outer kernel of the oat and is packed with fiber. It has a pleasant nutty flavor and is great if you need to boost your fiber intake. About a ¼ to ½ cup per smoothie is enough.

- ***Cocoa Powder*** – this helps to thicken the smoothie and is a great replacement for chocolate – in a banana smoothie, it makes it taste heavenly. Usually a couple of teaspoons will suffice.

- **Peanut Butter** – This is a multi-tasker of note. It can be a fat, a protein or a filler. 2 tablespoons is the maximum to add to a smoothie and do ensure that you get the sugar-free version.

- **Yoghurt, Avocado** – These all thicken the smoothie and act as good fillers.

Optional Extras

There are some optional extras that you might want to consider when making your smoothies – these can be used to enhance the flavor of the blend or to pack in more health benefits. As with the other items, do try and get the best quality possible. Here are some optional extras to consider:

- **Sweeteners** – I would suggest that you try your blend before adding sweeteners. Normally the fruit will sweeten it up more than enough. If you are using almond milk with the recipe I gave, the vanilla essence helps to enhance the flavor as well. That said, some smoothies need a bit of sweetness.

    Do try to go for natural sweeteners like stevia or maybe raw honey. Raw honey is a great anti-bacterial so can be a good choice. You could also use xylitol if you have it. Steer clear of artificial sweeteners like aspartame and never use pure granulated sugar.

- **Salt** – A lot has been said about how we take in too much salt in general. On this plan, the opposite is more likely to be true – by eating all-natural foods, you will not be getting much in the way of salt.

    Consider adding a pinch of salt to at least one of your smoothies every day. If you find that you start cramping, your body is asking you for more salt so increase your intake accordingly. You can use good old table salt or Himalayan Salt according to taste.

- **Kelp powder or Spirulina** – Seaweed has a range of nutrients but it is not necessarily something that you have access to on a daily basis. Adding a teaspoon or two of these to your smoothies helps you to get the benefits whilst masking the taste – they do not taste that great at all.

What to Expect from a Detox and How to Deal with the Symptoms

What you need to remember is that we tend to follow unhealthy lifestyles. Sugar and caffeine are two of the most common stimulants consumed today and there is a very good reason for that – they are highly addictive.

Ever noticed how difficult it is to stop at just one piece of chocolate or cake? That's because sugar acts on the same pleasure center in the brain that drugs do. If you were to look at a picture of your brain on crack, and then a picture of your brain on sugar, it would look the same.

Caffeine is not quite as bad but is still addictive. You are probably going to feel as though you are coming down with the flu and will find that your cravings increase initially.

The good news is that as you carry on going, you will find that the cravings also diminish and you will start to feel better and stronger. The only way to get through though is to stick to the plan strictly. Rest, drink enough water and do not cheat.

Here are some other common symptoms to expect:

- **Breakouts** – It has now been established that there is no link between the fat that you eat and acne. It has, however, been established that fluctuating blood sugar levels can have an impact on hormones and, consequently, on acne.

  During the first few days, your blood sugar is likely to fluctuate as your body gets used to the changes being made. This can cause your skin to breakout. This is normal and will not last long. As soon as your body adjusts, your skin will start to clear up again.

- **Flatulence and Bloating** – This is a very common symptom and is as a result of an increased fiber intake. You can try adding peppermint or fennel seeds into your smoothies to help with this. Again, this won't last long – once your body is used to the increased fiber intake, it will settle down again.

- **Constipation and/or Diarrhea** – Whilst not particularly present, this is again a reaction to the increased fiber intake. Again, it will only last a short while so do try to ride it out.

- **Brain Fog** – You are likely to feel as though you are in a bit of a stupor. This is generally because of withdrawal from caffeine and sugar. If this is a real problem for you, introduce a cup of green tea every morning and at lunch time – without milk or sugar.

  If this goes on for longer than 3 or 4 days, you need to re-evaluate what you are eating – you may not be getting enough calories, fat or protein overall.

- **Fatigue & Low Energy** – This is more a symptom of your body adjusting to the new way of doing things. Again, if this lasts more than 3 or 4 days, it is more likely a sign that you are not eating enough. Try to add an extra serving of protein to each meal and see if that helps.

- **Aches and Pains** – You are going to be surprised to hear this but there is very rarely a physical reason for developing aches and pains. Chances are that they are all in your head – literally. You need to remember that your body is not keen on changing the status quo.

  It is going to try all sorts of tricks to get you back to eating the way you were before. Think of these aches and pains as your body's way of throwing a temper tantrum. Again, this should only last a few days, until your body gets used to the new way of doing things.

- ***Cravings That Won't Quit*** – Your body can be compared to a toddler – it likes a set routine and will go to great lengths to get what it wants. It can send out some pretty strong cravings. The trick to dealing with these is to make sure that you are getting the right amount daily in terms of calories.

  You can also make adjustments to suit the palate – if your body is screaming for sugar, make sure that you have sweet fruit in your smoothie. If it wants something salty, add a little table salt. The main thing is to ensure that you do follow the plan exactly.

Once again, thank you for reading this book, and I hope you're getting a lot of valuable information. I would greatly appreciate it if you could take 30 seconds to leave me a review for this book on Amazon.com.

Chapter Five

Speed Up Your Weight Loss

Water Please

You should be drinking at least 8 glasses of water a day. That's 2 liters. This is even more vital when you are detoxifying. Getting enough water will help you to deal with the symptoms of detox more effectively.

Dehydration during detox is common and can lead to headaches and fatigue. Don't put yourself more at risk of feeling bad. The easiest way to ensure that you get enough is to have a bottle on hand with you at all times. If you see the bottle on the desk, it will remind you to drink the water.

Remember, you will need to drink 2 liters a day so measure how much water your bottle contains to figure out how many bottles you need to drink a day. And no, tea and coffee and smoothies do not count towards the total in this instance. Avoid commercial flavored waters – they tend to have a ton of sugar in them.

Drink your water! It doesn't matter if you do not feel thirsty – if you wait until you feel thirsty it means that you have already started to dehydrate. If you are not drinking enough water, the body retains what it has. This, in turn, makes it harder to flush out toxins.

The big benefit of drinking more water – you will find that you no longer feel as hungry – what we often feel as hunger pangs are actually a sign that we are dehydrated. Drink a glass of water if you are feeling hungry and it might just go away.

Goodnight Sweetheart

Are you one of those people that hits the snooze button over and over again or do you spring out of bed in the morning ready for the day? If you need to keep hitting the snooze button, there is a good chance that you are not getting enough sleep.

When you do not get enough sleep, your body is under stress and produces more cortisol. This, in turn, suppresses the hormones that control hunger and you end up eating more calories throughout the day.

The cure for not getting enough sleep is not hard – you simply need to get more. You can rationalize burning the candle at both ends as much as you want but there is no substitute for getting a full night's sleep.

You will feel more rested and be able to accomplish more after a proper night's rest. You owe it to yourself to make getting enough sleep a priority. You need to ensure that you get up at the same time every day, regardless of when you went to bed.

Work out the optimal time for you to wake up – you should be up and about at least an hour before you need to leave for work. Now work out your bedtime – it should be at least 8 hours before you need to get up. Give yourself about 15 minutes to fall asleep.

Give yourself about an hour before bedtime to wind down and relax so that your body starts to prepare for sleep. This means switching off the TV, your computer and your laptop and doing something that will not stimulate your mind to much in the interim.

In the morning, climb out of bed and open the curtains immediately. According to findings published in Women's Health Magazine, the simple act increasing the amount of exposure to early morning light will decrease the risk of being overweight.

It's not that hard once you get used to it. Try this experiment – pretend that there is a power blackout and don't switch on any lights, etc. for one night.

Use candles instead. You'll be amazed at how early you start to become tired. It just goes to show how much artificial light stimulates the mind.

If you are doing the smoothie cleanse, your 7-8 hours of sleep a day becomes even more vital – your body needs the time to really repair and to clear out all the toxins. You will also find, especially during the first few days, that you are going to be more tired.

If you battle to fall asleep at night, you can try the following:

- Keep a notepad and pen next to the bed – if anything is worrying you, write it down and you can deal with it in the morning.

- Add lettuce to your evening smoothie – lettuce induces calm and has a soporific effect.

- Practice good sleep hygiene – block out as much light as possible, block out as much noise as possible and try to keep the room at an even, cool temperature.

Warm Water and Lemon Juice

Now that you are up, have a glass of tepid water with lemon juice in it. It is better to use fresh lemon juice if you are able – not only is it more nutritious but it is more palatable. Use the juice of either a half or whole lemon in a whole glass of water.

Lemon water taken in this way will stimulate the detox process, help with digestion, boost immunity, help clear out uric acid, stimulate the mind, reduce inflammation and start the body burning fat and also give you a dose of Vitamin C.

The question is not so much why you should adopt this habit but why you haven't already.

Stretch

You know how to stretch; just do it. Your body loves stretching. If you want, learn a few yoga postures that will help. It really doesn't matter as long as you are elongating the muscles.

Stretching for as little as 5 minutes every morning will help to tone and smooth the muscles in your body; boost circulation and lymph drainage and help you to feel calmer and more relaxed.

Now Move!

I did say that there was no intense exercise program here. There is, however, some exercise. Every morning, before your morning smoothie, you need to do around 15-30 minutes of cardio. You could walk, cycle, jog – whatever you want, and are able, to do.

If you are a bit of a couch potato, start off slowly. Walk for 5 minutes or 10 minutes. Build it up as your go along. By the end of the 9 days, you'll find that you look forward to your exercise time. Even a five-minute walk helps to boost energy levels and gets the heart pumping.

It will help to reduce feelings of anxiety, depression and stress. It will also help you deal with the symptoms of detox. Moving is what the body was designed to do. Get moving, even if it is just a little.

Best of all, it speeds up the weight loss benefit of this plan. You do not need to kill yourself exercising – even walking around the block a few times will be beneficial.

Put Your Back into It

Strength training is another vital component here – again, you need not kill yourself but do incorporate some strength training at least every second day. You don't even have to buy special exercise equipment – look in your grocery cupboards at home if you're desperate – a can of baked beans can double as a dumbbell, at least, initially.

Get creative and you'll soon find that there are plenty of "weights" that you can use in your own home. This is going to be the key to losing the maximum amount of weight possible because it will help you to turn that flab into muscles.

The reason that you are not able to maintain the weight lost during one of those fad diets (Remember the Cabbage Soup Diets?) is that the body is, in essence, starving for nutrients and starts to use muscle mass. You may lose some weight initially but you also lose muscle mass.

And muscle mass is essential for anyone trying to lose weight – even when muscle is at rest, it still burns more energy than fat does.

More muscle = Better fat-burning potential.

That also translates into better energy all the time.

Extra Nutrients

You will also need to take a multi-vitamin every morning. Whilst this plan is going to really improve the nutritional content of your diet, it is still going to be difficult to get all the vitamins and minerals that you optimally need.

Studies have found that those who are deficient in nutrients are more at risk of being overweight so it is better to ensure that you have enough. You are more likely to overeat if your body is nutrient deficient. You do NOT need to take mega-doses. A simple multi-vitamin supplement will do.

In addition, unless you are eating oily fish twice a week, you are going to need to take a fish oil supplement. And, yes, it has to be fish oil – our bodies are not able to process the Omega-3s in plants.

Omega-3s are essential to the body – that is why they are called essential fatty acids. They are used in a range of processes but the most important benefit is that they reduce inflammation. Omega-3's can help to protect us from developing depression, heart disease, high LDL cholesterol, degenerative conditions like arthritis and dementia.

It also changes the way in which the body uses its fat stores – it encourages the burning of fats and triglycerides and prevents the body from storing the visceral fat (belly fat) that is so dangerous in terms of health.

There is one more supplement that may be necessary if you are not going to use yoghurt or kefir – a probiotic supplement. Studies have linked visceral fat – the fat stored around the abdomen with decreased levels of the healthy bacteria in the gut. The aim here is to re-populate your gut with healthy bacteria.

Get Family and Friends Involved

It will be important to explain the plan to family and friends so that they can support you – eating out socially is going to be difficult to accomplish and your friends and family need to know what is going on.

Be prepared for all the "good" advice and also be prepared for some negative statements. There has been a lot of misinformation spread about smoothies in the past and a lot of people still think that smoothies are fattening. This eating plan is based on real results and is healthy. What gave smoothies a bad rap was that people were piling in the fruit, etc. and adding in too much sugar, without enough protein.

I once saw a recipe for a smoothie that was basically just banana and condensed milk mixed in with water. It was practically pure sugar but was being billed as a healthy fruit smoothie. The idea that smoothies are bad for you is also based on outdated science and theories.

We now know that it is the effect of the food on our blood sugar that is more important than the actual amount of calories or fat that the food contains.

As recently as 15 years ago, we were told that we must stick to a low-fat diet but that sugar was okay because it contained no fat. This has since been disproved but attitudes in general take longer than that to adjust.

Let your family know that you are not going to be yourself for the first few days and enlist their support in relation to the household chores and cooking and cleaning.

You can also mention the fact that you are on this eating plan to colleagues at work if you want to. It is important to have a good support structure in place when changing the way you do things as a rule. Someone to talk to when it seems easier to break the rules is a very important part of making this work.

Choose someone that will offer real support though and not try to force their views on healthy eating onto you as well.

Your New Bath Time Ritual

For the first three nights, you are going to support the detox process by having an Epsom salt bath. After the first week, you can reduce that to two days a week.

Warning: If you suffer from high blood pressure, leave this section out completely.

You have no doubt seen advertisements for Magnesium oils and sprays that allow you to get your daily dose of Magnesium through the skin. Science has proven that Magnesium can be absorbed efficiently through the skin or taken from the diet.

You are now going to benefit from that knowledge, without paying the hefty price tag for the fancy magnesium oils and sprays. All you need is good old-fashioned Epsom Salts.

Epsom Salts are made up of Magnesium and Sulfate. All you need to do to get the benefit is to put about two cups of Epsom Salts in the bath tub and add hot water. Soak for at least 15 minutes.

Keep a big glass of water next to the bath and sip frequently. The water should be at room temperature and should not have any ice in it.

I have an Epsom Salt bath two to three times a week – I soak for at least half an hour. I take a good book with me and I find that it is really relaxing.

Find some way for you to relax in the bath – maybe this means reading a book or magazine or simply lying back listening to music. Do whatever works for you in this instance.

I also add:

- 5-6 drops Juniper essential oil
- 5-6 drops Eucalyptus essential oil
- 5-6 drops Sweet Orange essential oil

The oils are not essential but they do help to increase the benefits of the bath. Juniper is good for promoting circulation; Eucalyptus for easing aching muscles and Sweet Orange is good for pepping you up. I chose these oils because they do not interfere with me sleeping. They help you feel refreshed but not over-stimulated.

Give yourself a vigorous rubdown with your towel afterwards to further the effects. Do this at least an hour before bed to promote better sleep. Do have a warm blanket on your bed – your body temperature will, at first, be raised but will soon lower again.

You must NOT consume the salts internally. Unless you are under the supervision of a properly licensed and qualified health care practitioner, it is a really bad idea to consume the salts internally. They can have a profound laxative effect if taken internally.

If you have very sore muscles, you can also make a paste of Epsom salts to apply. Mix the salts with at enough water to make a stiff paste and apply to the sore area, leave for at least 20 minutes before rinsing off. Do not do this if the skin is broken – it will burn a lot.

Don't apply any lotions or creams of any sort to the skin after this bath – the body needs to sweat to get rid of the toxins and creams will end up getting in the way and clogging the pores.

The Health Benefits of Epsom Salts

- ***Relax and relieve stress*** – During your bath, the body will absorb the magnesium it needs. Magnesium is essential for the production of serotonin. This process encourages the production of serotonin and your mind and body feel more relaxed. The body only absorbs what it needs so there is no danger of overdosing on magnesium.

- ***Relieves Aching Muscles*** – Relaxing in the tub of Epsom Salts will also relax aching muscles. This is perfect for those who are suffering through detox. The full benefit is felt the next day, however, because you will have had a better night's rest.

- **Boost Circulation and Metabolism** – This is great for getting your circulation moving and revving up your metabolism. Your blood pressure will be elevated whilst soaking so you should avoid this treatment if you have high blood pressure.

- **Magnesium is Essential** – Magnesium is vital to the body's nervous and musculature systems. Absorption through the skin has been proven to be the most effective means to get sufficient quantities of Magnesium. Magnesium is also vital for those wanting to lose weight – it helps the body increase the effectiveness of insulin.

- **Softer Skin** – Magnesium is great for the skin as well. Your skin will feel a lot softer when you get out of the bath.

- **It Detoxes the Body** – An Epsom Salt bath will help to pull toxins out of the body. This process doesn't end in the bath.

You may find that you feel quite warm after the bath – this is normal as your body is still detoxing. The Epsom Salts also encourage the release of toxins during sweating after the bath – it is important to note, however, that despite the increased sweating, you may still feel cold. Be prepared for that.

Enjoying this book?

Check out my other best sellers!

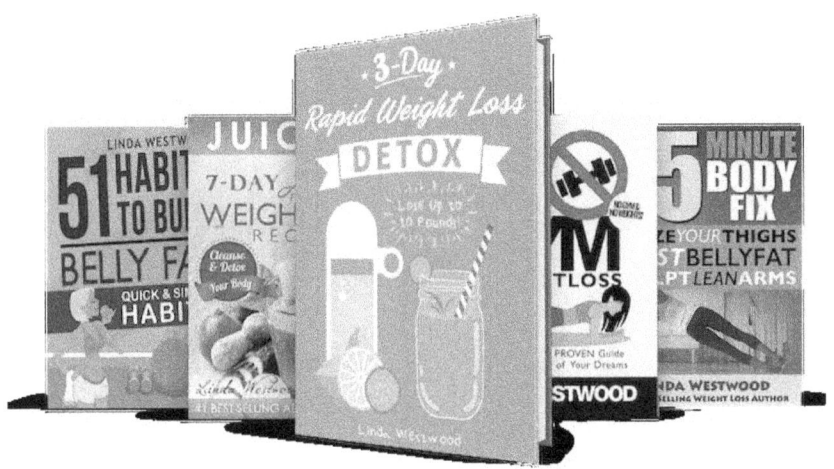

Get your next book on sale here:

TopFitnessAdvice.com/go/books

Chapter Six

Long-Term Weight Loss

The beauty of this plan is that you only need to stick to it for nine days. It is not recommended that you continue for longer than this. You will now no doubt be fired up and looking for ways to keep the "buzz" going.

The good news is that you have now broken some of your bad eating habits and have seen the astonishing benefits that come from eating in this manner.

For optimal benefits, it is a good idea to slowly start transitioning back to a more "normal" diet.

Here are some ideas to help you along that journey:

- Your system has had no solid foods over the last nine days so you want to ease back into things slowly. Start by introducing one light meal a day in place of one of the smoothies.

- This meal should consider mostly of raw vegetables and should be a light meal. You also need to add in some protein. Smoked chicken, steamed fish, salmon or boiled eggs are a good way to keep the meal light and healthy.

- Keep the food simple – add flavor with spices rather than with creamy and rich sauces.

- After a week or so, you can start swopping out your second smoothie for a meal – again, keep to simple foods.

- After a week like this, you can swop out the last smoothie if you want to. Many people opt to leave at least one meal as a smoothie a day – it helps with energy and is convenient.

A Healthy Diet

If you go back to eating as you were before, you will simply start to feel sick and will start to gain weight again. It makes no sense to fall back into bad habits. Fortunately, your body now has a taste for the healthy food and it will want more of the same.

Make sure that you have a diet rich in raw fruit and vegetables and eat protein at every meal to further your weight loss goals. Try to follow a whole food approach when looking at what foods to buy - was the food made by nature or made by a factory? Highly processed foods have few, if any nutrients and should be avoided as far as possible.

You should also have learned that healthy food does not need to be bland and boring. Use the herbs and spices that you have learned about here in cooking. Look into making herbal teas to continue the detox process more gently – Fennel, for example, is an excellent diuretic.

Parsley tea is a blood cleanser and bone builder. Cumin tea will help ease digestive upsets. Alfalfa tea is alkalizing. The list goes on and on - do yourself a favor and look into herbal teas and what they can do for you.

Just remember, you should not take a herbal tea for longer than 10 days in a row. Take a break for about a week and start up again if you want to. At the very least, you need to maintain your 3 cups of green tea a day. Try livening it up a bit with mint or lemon or get adventurous and add a bit of cumin or nutmeg.

You should still be drinking your lemon juice in warm water every morning – kick that up a few notches by adding a ¼ teaspoon cinnamon (to regulate blood sugar) and a ¼ teaspoon cayenne pepper (to rev up your metabolism).

I'm not going to lie – it does not taste that great but you do get used to the taste pretty quickly, so hang in there.

If you really and truly find that you cannot get used to the taste, have plain lemon water again and mix the cayenne pepper and cinnamon to a teaspoon of honey and take it like that. It helps it taste a little sweeter.

Exercise

You would have begun your exercise program during the smoothie cleanse and you need to continue with it. Set yourself exercise goals as you go along so that you do push yourself to do better.

Get someone to exercise with you and you will motivate each other to do better. Consider signing up for some sort of marathon so that you have something to train for.

Stretching

Carry on with your stretching exercises, they are important for keeping your joints supple and will help with mobility later in life. Stretching will continue to maintain the tone in the muscles and help the lymphatic and circulatory systems to work as well as they should.

A warm-up is essential before any workout to reduce the risks of injuring your muscles. You could also incorporate a basic five-minute stretching routine before bed time to help you to ease the stress and tension of the day and to release sore muscles.

Cardio

This can be painless – let's say that you walk for 5 minutes a day and manage one block. Next week, set your goal for two blocks.

When you can manage two blocks in 5 minutes, add another block, and so on. You need to aim to work up to at least 15-30 minutes of cardio a day in order to keep your heart healthy.

Try to find exercises that you enjoy doing so that you keep them up. Anything that gets your heart rate up is considered cardio. You want to exercise at about 80% to 85% of your maximum heart rate in order to burn fat. You calculate your maximum heart rate by subtracting your age from 220 and work from there.

Take your resting pulse rate from time to time when you get up in the morning. Simply set your timer for 10 seconds and then count the number of heartbeats during that time. Multiply this total by 6 and you will know what your resting heart rate is.

As you start to get fitter, your heart rate will slow down. Trained athletes have heart rates in the range of 40 to 60 beats per minute. It can be a valuable exercise to record this rate once a week and monitor your progress overall.

Strength Training

Learn how to strength train properly so that you can get a body that really looks shapely with muscles that are strong and not flabby.

You can buy a basic set of weights quite inexpensively and there are tons of workouts that you can find online. Alternatively, buy yourself a DVD or join a gym. You can also set up a couple of sessions with a personal trainer to help set a proper routine for you.

When it comes to strength training, it is important to get the moves right so that you reduce the risk of injury and undue strain on the muscles. Strength training is important when it comes to building bone density and fighting the weight gain that comes with advancing age.

Don't Forget the Smoothies

Some people opt to have smoothies for breakfast or lunch, even after they've gone back to "normal" eating habits. I think that this is a great way to boost energy levels and to carry on nourishing your body. Just stick to the same healthy principles that you read here.

You can, of course, do the smoothie cleanse at any time you want to – it is advisable to give yourself a break for at least two weeks before starting your next cleanse but there is nothing stopping you from scheduling regular cleanses in order to further boost weight loss or when you feel that you need it.

You are, at some point or another, going to hit a plateau when it comes to weight loss and the smoothie cleanse can help you to get over that and lose that next bit of weight.

Smoothies for Healing

Smoothies are great for immune boosting – when you are feeling ill you hardly feel like cooking or much like eating – use any of the smoothie recipes in this book when you are ill in place of meals and they will give you an amazing immune boost.

Smoothies are actually a lot healthier for you than soup is – it's amazing that chicken soup is still considered the top food for clearing up colds and flu.

Others who are considering purchasing this book would love to know what you think. If you could spare a few seconds, they would greatly appreciate reading an honest review from you. Simply visit the page on Amazon.com.

Chapter Seven

Breakfast Smoothies

Green is for Go

Breakfast is the most important meal of the day – it gets your metabolism revved up and helps you with the energy that you need for the day ahead. Smoothie breakfast suit just about everyone and are a blessing if you can't face eating first thing in the morning.

Your mornings will become routine – get up and greet the sun; have your lemon juice in water; stretch and exercise; and then prepare the smoothie. Every morning for breakfast, you are going to have a green smoothie. This is vital. It is what makes this program work.

Start with the basic green smoothie detailed below. The ingredients have been specially chosen to increase detoxification and boost energy. The ingredients do work well together so it has a fresh taste.

Take some time in the morning to relax and sip the smoothie. Gulping it down will increase your chances of swallowing air with it and that, in turn, leads to bloating and discomfort. Give yourself at least 15 minutes and sit down to drink your smoothie.

The chlorophyll content of the leaves is a life-giving force – literally. It is what plants survive on. You can benefit by taking in this energy yourself. You will get a major boost from your green smoothie and the energy will last until lunchtime.

Green smoothies rev up the metabolism and help to flush toxins out of the body. Here are some basic green smoothie recipes to start you off:

Basic Green Smoothie

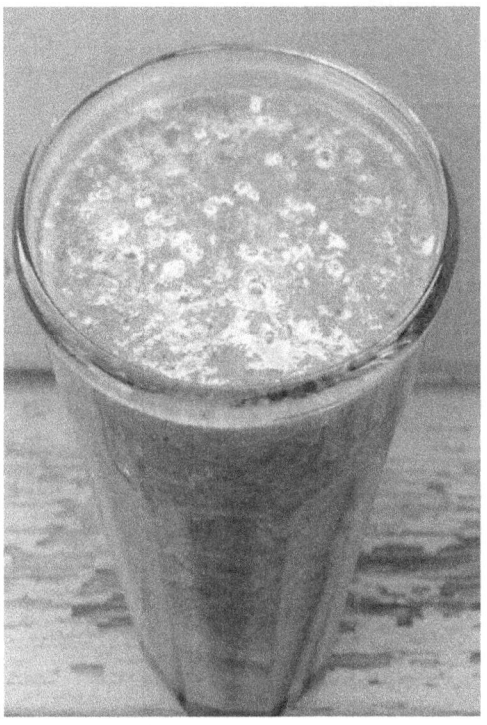

(Serves 1)

Ingredients

- 1 apple, chopped up
- The juice of 1 lemon
- 1 cup kale
- 1 stalk of celery
- 1/3 cup flat leaf parsley, cilantro or detoxifying herb of your choice
- 1 tablespoon ground pumpkin seeds
- 1 tablespoon chia seeds or a serving of whey protein powder

- 1 teaspoon fennel seeds, crushed
- 1/4 teaspoon ground cinnamon
- 1 1/4 cups chilled almond milk
- 1 tablespoon fresh peppermint (Optional)
- 1/3 cup fresh wheatgrass (Sprout your own, if possible)
- 1 teaspoon turmeric
- ½ cup sprouts of your choice

Directions

1. If applicable, soak Chia seeds for at least an hour before adding to smoothie. Whizz everything up in the blender until smooth. Serve it as is, or over ice.

Kiwi Kale Smoothie

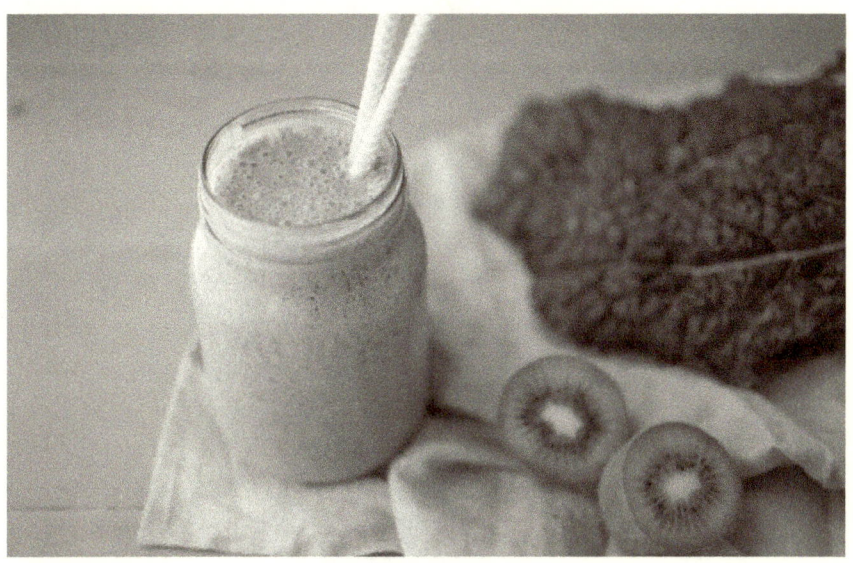

(Serves 2)

Ingredients

- 2 kiwi, peeled and halved
- ½ banana, peeled
- 1 cup kale
- ½ cup Greek yoghurt
- 2 tablespoons ground flax seed or sunflower seed
- ½ cup apple juice
- 10 ice cubes

Directions

1. Whizz everything up in the blender until smooth. Serve it as is, or over ice.

Ginger Mint Smoothie

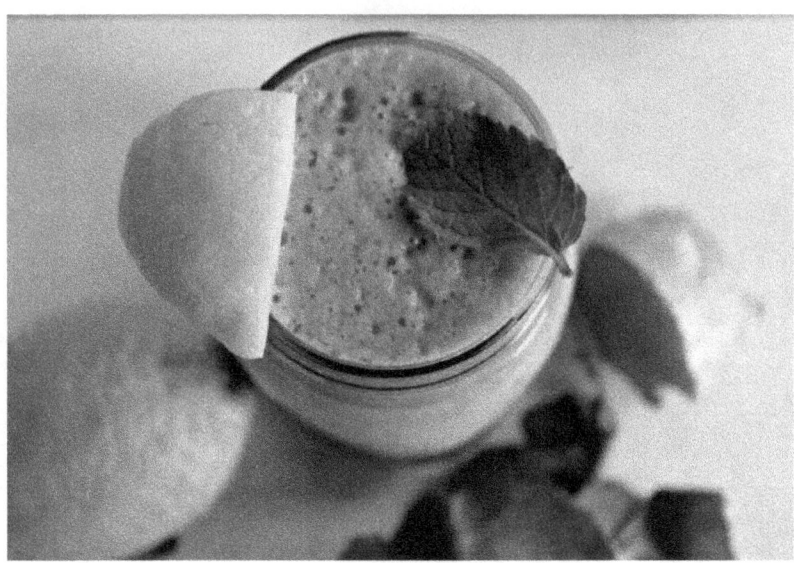

(Serves 1)

Ingredients

- 1 handful spinach
- 1 handful mint
- 1 handful parsley
- Juice of half a lemon
- 1/2 a cucumber
- 1 large celery stalk
- 1 inch piece of fresh ginger

Directions

1. Whizz everything up in the blender until smooth. Serve it as is, or over ice.

Orange and Avo Smoothie

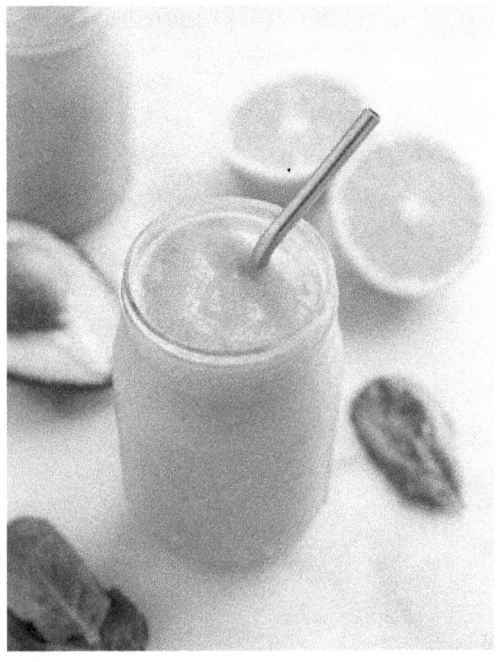

(Serves 1)

Ingredients

- 1 cup kale or baby spinach
- 1 large orange or a couple of Satsuma's, peeled
- 1/3 cup parsley
- 1/2 small avocado
- 1/2 cup apple, chopped
- 1 cup coconut milk or milk of your choice, chilled
- 1/2 cup ice
- 1 tablespoon lemon juice
- ¼ teaspoon cayenne pepper

Directions

1. Whizz everything up in the blender until smooth. Serve it as is, or over ice.

The Green Monster

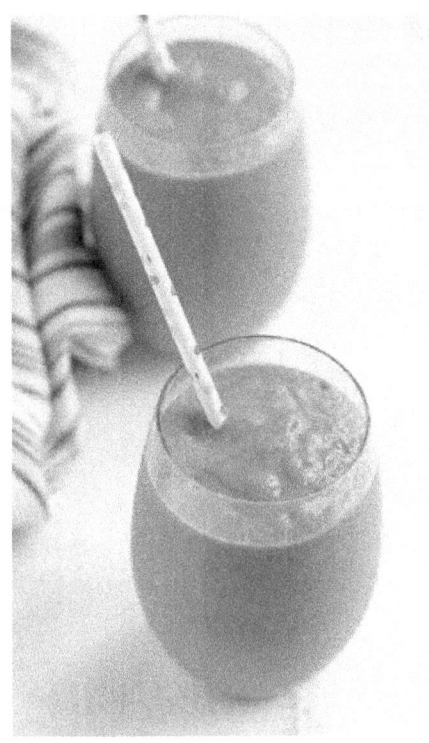

(Serves 1)

Ingredients

- 4 celery stalks
- 1 cucumber
- 1 cup kale
- ½ green apple
- ½ lime
- 1 tablespoon coconut oil
- ½ cup almond milk
- 1 cup pineapple

- 1 tablespoon turmeric
- ¼ teaspoon cayenne pepper
- 3 or 4 black peppercorns

Directions

1. Whizz everything up in the blender until smooth. Serve it as is or over ice.

Sprout Smoothie

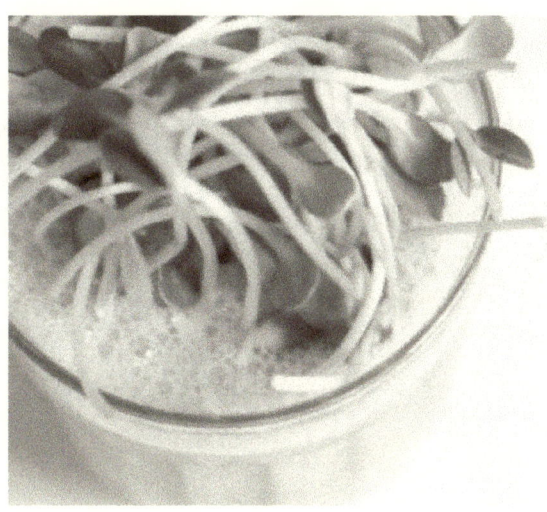

(Serves 1)

Ingredients

- 1 cup wheatgrass or sunflower greens
- 1 cup alfalfa or other a leafy sprout of your choosing
- 1 cup leafy greens--spinach, kale, etc. tightly packed
- 1 carrot
- 1 apple
- 1 orange
- 1 cup almond milk
- ½ cup oat bran

Directions

1. Blend everything together until smooth. Add more almond milk if you want a more liquid texture.

Eastern Delight Smoothie

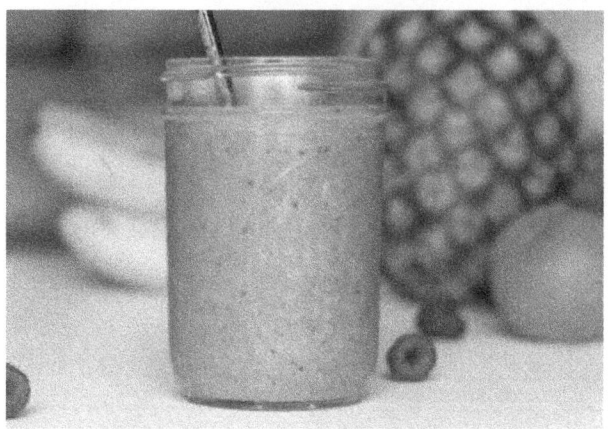

(Serves 2)

Ingredients

- 1 apple
- 2 cups cold almond milk
- 2 tablespoons coconut flakes
- 1 ripe banana, peeled
- 2 persimmons (remove the stem and top and then quarter – you can eat the skin)
- ½ cup frozen pineapple chunks
- 2 handfuls of kale
- ¼ cup sprouts
- Ice to taste

Directions

1. Blend all ingredients until smooth. The persimmon is a much-loved fruit in Near Eastern cultures and has a

wonderful sweet flavor. The skin is the nicest part - so don't peel it. The fruit is packed with anti-oxidants and vitamin C.

Apple, Mint and Cucumber Summer Smoothie

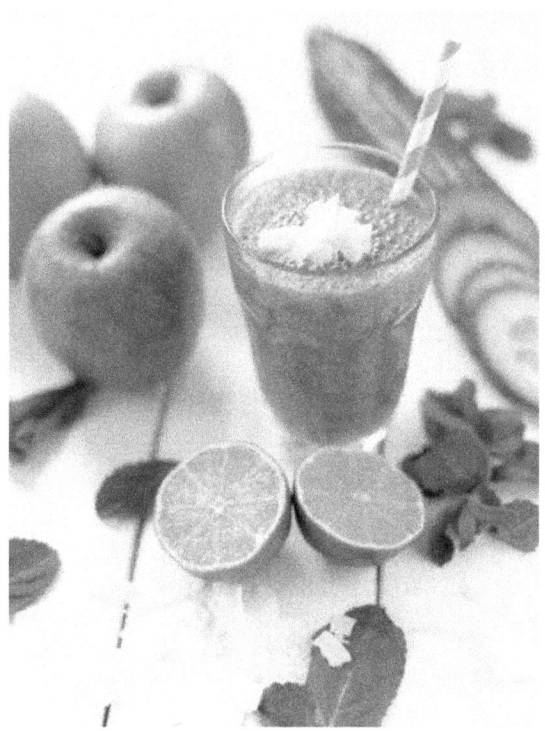

(Serves 2)

Ingredients

- 1 cup cucumber – chopped
- 2 apples
- 1/4 cup cold almond milk
- 1/4 cup chopped fresh mint
- ½ cup plain oatmeal (not instant)
- ¼ cup sunflower seeds

- ¼ borage flowers (reserve some to decorate if you want to)
- 10 ice cubes

Directions

1. Add all ingredients and blend well until smooth, adding ice cubes two at a time. The borage flowers have a taste similar to that of the cucumber and are rich in omega 3s, calcium and potassium. They make a lovely garnish as well.

Green Tea Mango Delight

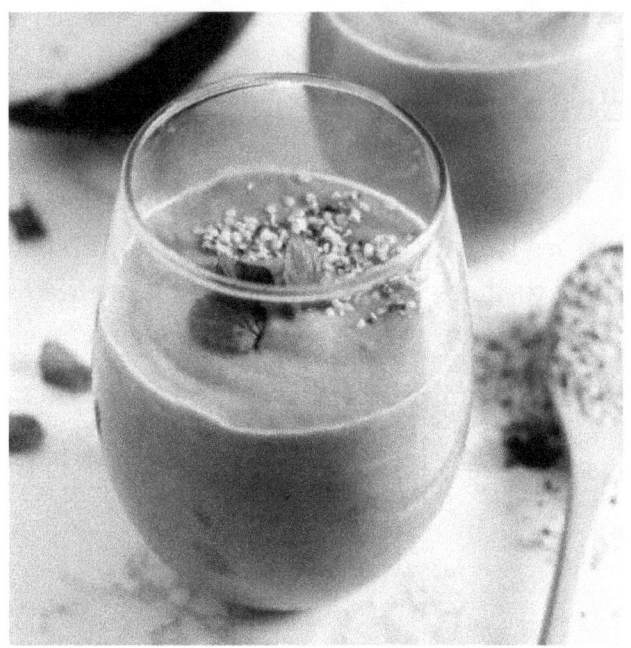

(Serves 1)

Ingredients

- 1 cup green tea
- 1 cup fresh or frozen mango chunks
- 1/2 medium avocado
- 1 cup kale
- 1/2 tablespoon coconut oil
- 1/3 cup parsley
- A dash of sea salt
- A little honey or stevia, if required

Directions

1. Whizz everything up in the blender until smooth. Serve it as is or over ice.

Mean Green Fat Buster

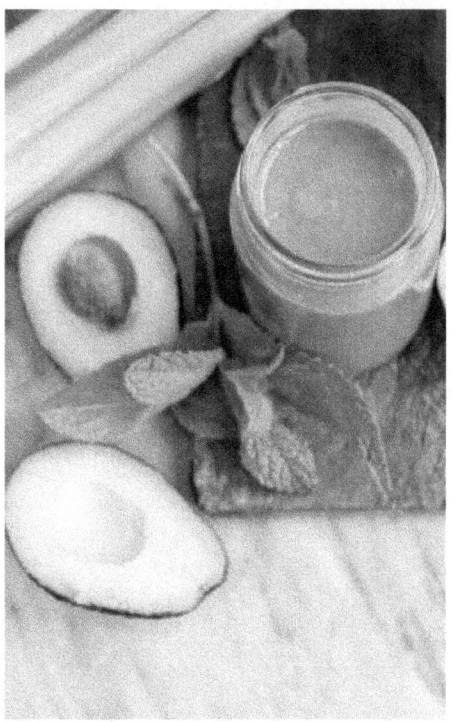

(Serves 1)

Ingredients

- 1 cup milk of choice or water
- 1 fresh or frozen medium banana
- 1/2 cup frozen blueberries
- 1 cup kale
- 1 teaspoon honey to sweeten
- ½ cup wheatgrass
- ½ avocado or 1 tablespoon of coconut oil
- 4 sprigs of celery

- 1/3 cup of fennel

Directions

1. Whizz everything up in the blender until smooth. Serve it as is or over ice.

Fruits of the Sea Recipe

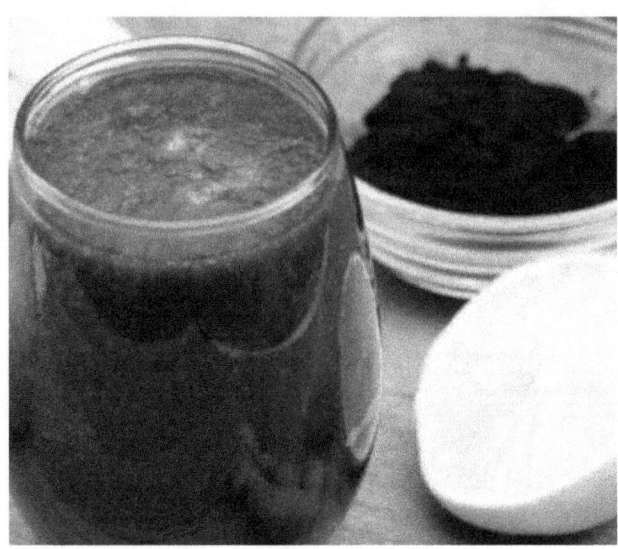

(Serves 1)

Ingredients

- 1 cup almond milk
- Juice of 1/2 lemon
- 1 cup kale
- 1 teaspoon spirulina
- 14 almonds
- 1/2 tablespoon honey
- 3-5 ice cubes (optional)
- 1/4 cup cilantro
- 1/4 cup arugula
- Juice of 1/2 lime
- 1/2 cup fresh or frozen pineapple or mango chunks

Directions

1. Whizz everything up in the blender until smooth. Serve it as is or over ice. This tastes very fresh and green – the pineapple removes that bitter edge and the lime rounds off the flavor.

Tropical Heat

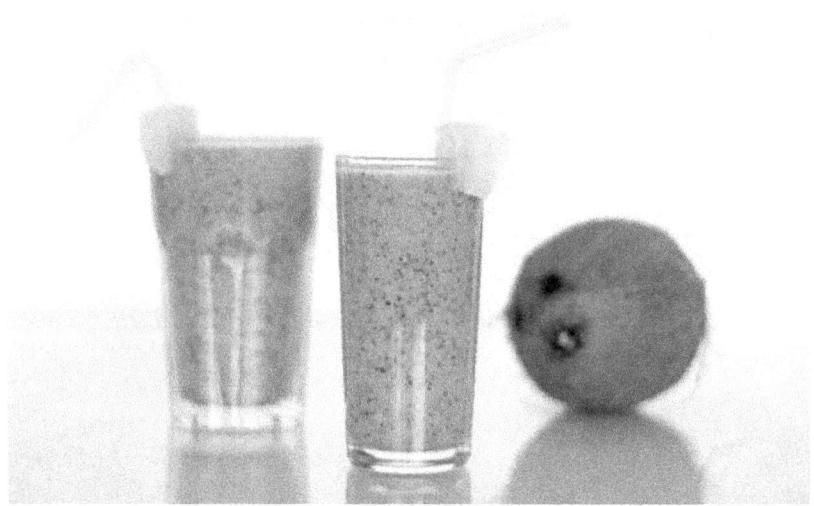

(Serves 2)

Ingredients

- 2 cups kale
- 2 cups coconut milk
- 2 cups pineapple
- 1 cup mango
- Juice of ½ lemon
- 1 tablespoon fresh ginger
- 1 tablespoon turmeric
- 4 or 5 black peppercorns
- 14 almonds

Directions

1. Whizz everything up in the blender until smooth. Serve it as is or over ice. The ginger and black pepper may seem like a strange mix with the fruits but they all combine for a flavor that is deliciously different.

Beet Cleansing Smoothie

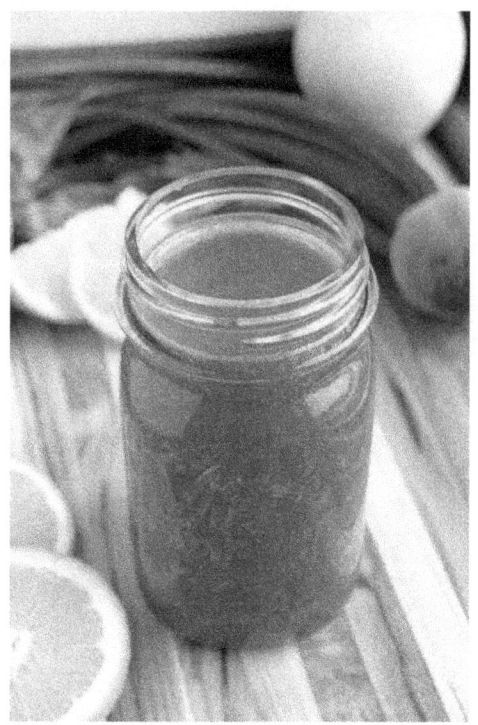

(Serves 2)

Ingredients

- 2 cups beet greens or chard
- 1 cup coconut water
- 2 oranges, peeled
- 1 small raw beet, peeled
- Juice of ½ lemon
- 1 tablespoon Chia seeds
- 1 tablespoon coconut oil

Directions

1. Peeling the beet when raw is a little tougher than when it is cooked but it does get rid of that taste of dirt that the outer layer often has. Whizz everything up in the blender until smooth. Serve it as is or over ice.

Chapter Eight

Lunch Smoothies

Most of us tend to eat lunch on the run – the beauty of smoothies is that they are quick and easy to drink. If you're at work, store your smoothie in the fridge until lunchtime.

Better yet, if you could take your blender to work, you could make the smoothies fresh there.

If taking your smoothie to work is not a possibility, try to find a place near your office that makes smoothies.

Speak to them about what you'd like them to put in yours. They may be willing to accommodate you.

If you are going to try this option, do make sure that they use fresh fruits, etc. and not a smoothie powdered mix, or a combination of the two – many companies do use the powder and then throw in some bits of blitzed fruit and ice to improve the texture.

It is best not to store the smoothie overnight. If you make too much or can't get to your smoothie at lunch, you can freeze it for a later time.

Don't be alarmed if the color of the smoothie changes in the freezer – it does not mean that it has gone bad.

Red Berry Ginger Zinger

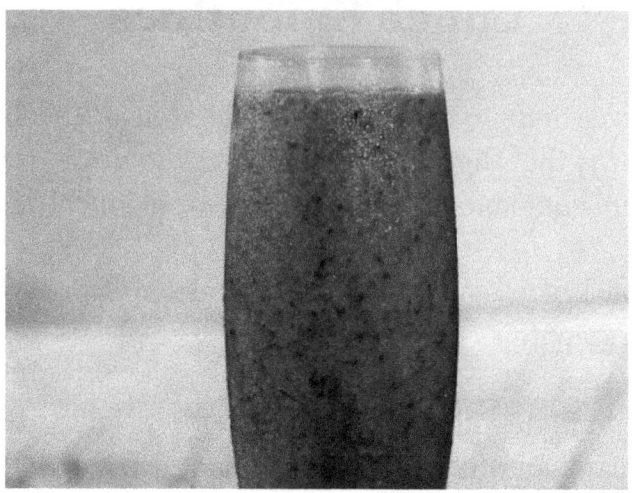

(Serves 2)

Ingredients

- 1 cup raspberries, frozen
- ¾ cup chilled milk of your choice
- 1 ½ tablespoon honey
- 2 teaspoons fresh ginger, grated
- 1 teaspoon each of flaxseed and pumpkin seed, ground
- 2 teaspoons lemon juice
- 1 tablespoon coconut oil

Directions

1. Put all the ingredients into the blender and whizz up until smooth.

Bring on the Beans Smoothie

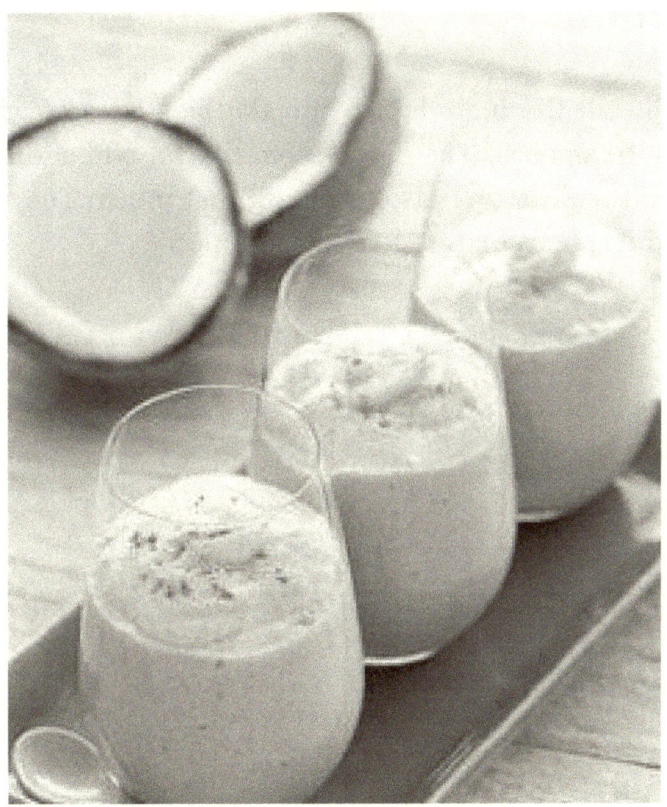

(Serves 1)

Ingredients

- 1¼ cup almond or rice milk
- ⅔ cup white beans, rinsed
- 1½ cups mango, frozen or fresh
- 1/3 cup mint
- 1 tablespoon coconut oil
- 1/3 cup fresh coconut

- Ice if required

Directions

1. Put all the ingredients into the blender and whizz up until smooth. The beans seem like an odd addition but you really won't taste them all that much. They do add quite a nice texture to the smoothie.

Vegetarian Smoothie

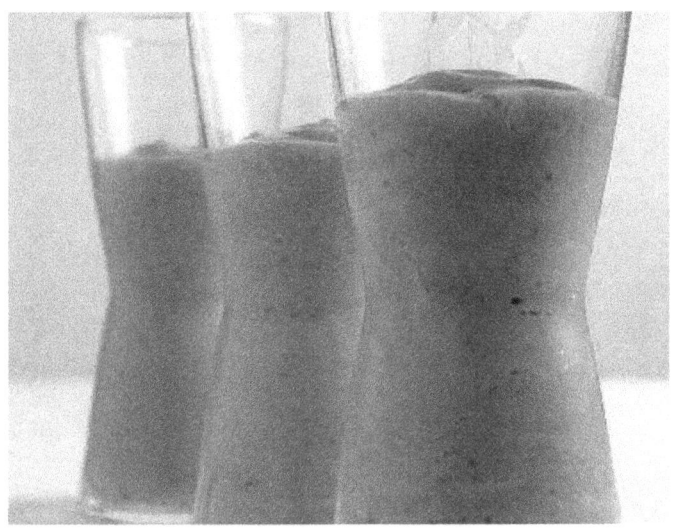

(Serves 2)

Ingredients

- 1 cup frozen mixed berries
- 1/2 cup grapes
- 1 tablespoon honey
- Banana, peeled
- 1 cup tofu
- Water or ice to taste

Directions

1. Put all the ingredients into the blender and whizz up until smooth. Tofu makes a nice protein rich option for the vegetarian.

Got a Date Smoothie

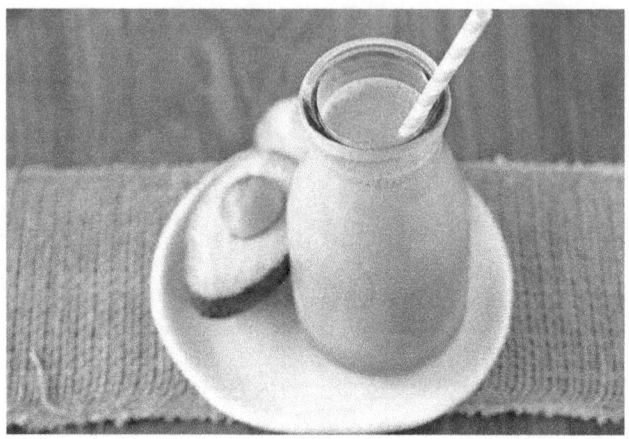

(Serves 1)

Ingredients

- 1 cup milk of your choice
- ½ avocado, frozen for a bit more texture
- 1 tablespoon cocoa powder
- 4 large soft dates
- Dash of cinnamon
- 1 teaspoon vanilla extract
- 1 T. raw nut butter of your choice
- Pinch of sea salt
- 5 ice cubes

Directions

1. Put all the ingredients into the blender and whizz up until smooth.

Awesome Melon Smoothie

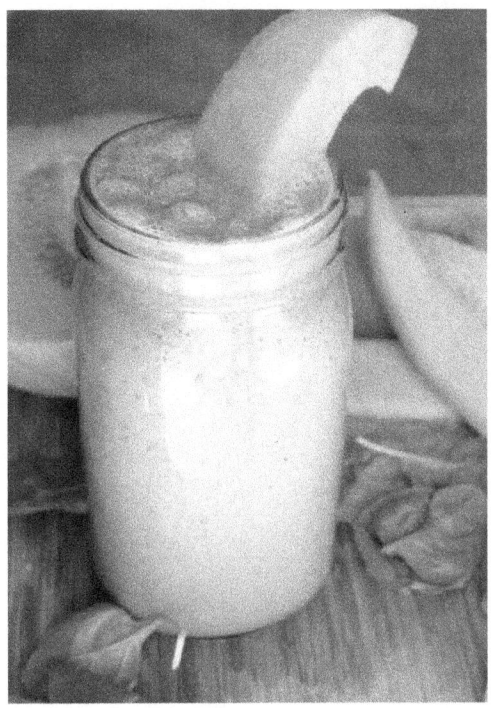

(Serves 2)

Ingredients

- 1 cup almond milk
- 1 cup cucumber
- 1 cup frozen cantaloupe
- 1/2 banana
- 2 cups kale
- 1 tablespoon flaxseeds
- 1 tablespoon chia seeds
- 1 teaspoon cinnamon

- 1 teaspoon pure vanilla extract
- 1/2 teaspoon peppermint extract
- 14 almonds
- 4 – 6 ice cubes
- Splash of water to taste

Directions

1. Put all the ingredients into the blender and whizz up until smooth.

Kefir Smoothie

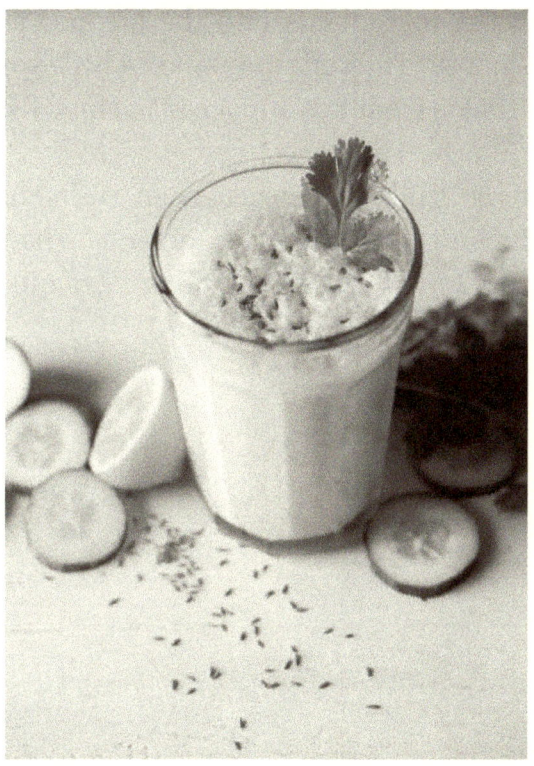

(Serves 2)

Ingredients

- 2 cups unsweetened whole milk kefir, chilled
- 1 cup chopped cucumber
- 1/4 cup fresh mint leaves
- Juice of 1 lemon
- 1/4 teaspoon ground cumin
- Pinch of salt

Directions

1. Put all the ingredients into the blender and whizz up until smooth. The kefir may smell a little sour but that it fine – that is what it is supposed to smell like.

2. All it is milk that has been fermented by the introduction of a strain of bacteria – bacteria that is necessary for the healthy functioning of our guts.

Anti-Oxidant Overload

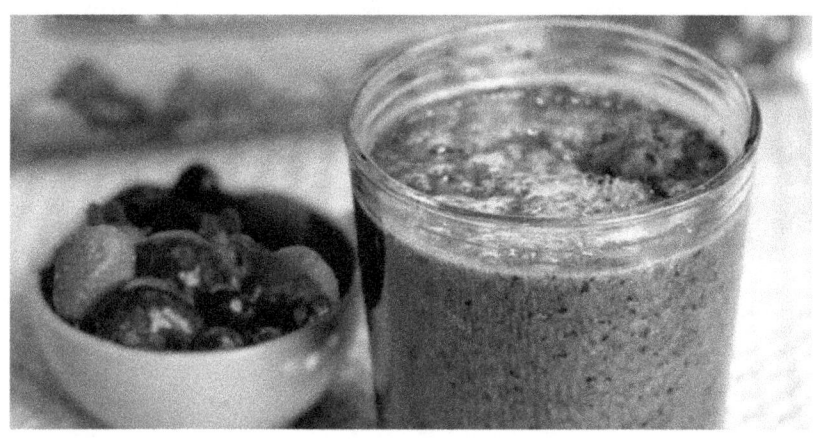

(Serves 1)

Ingredients

- 1/4 cup frozen or fresh blueberries
- 1/4 cup frozen or fresh raspberries
- 1/4 cup frozen or fresh strawberries
- 1/4 cup kale
- 1 cup almond milk
- 14 almonds
- ¼ teaspoon cinnamon
- 1 tablespoon turmeric
- 4 or 5 black peppercorns
- ¼ cup oat bran

Directions

1. Put all the ingredients into the blender and whizz up until smooth. When looking to increase the anti-oxidant punch of a smoothie, always remember, the more colors the better.

Mint and Watermelon Refresher

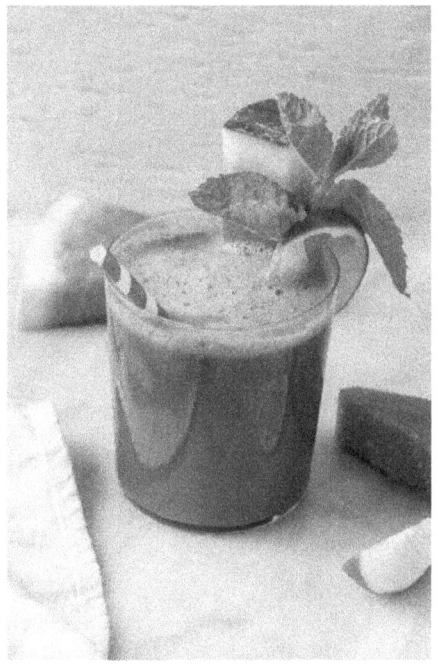

(Serves 1)

Ingredients

- 1/2 cucumber
- 1 1/2 cups frozen watermelon
- 1/3 cup loose fresh mint leaves
- 1/2 lime, juiced
- ½ cup raspberries
- 1 cup coconut water
- ½ avocado
- Water as needed for blending

Directions

1. Blend well and serve immediately.

Almond Milk and Berry Recipe

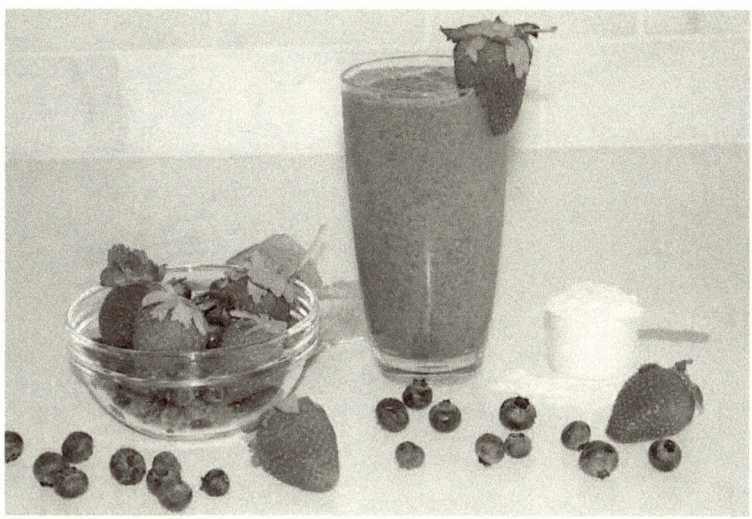

(Serves 2)

Ingredients

- ½ a medium sized banana, peeled and sliced
- ¼ cup blueberries – frozen or fresh
- ¼ cup strawberries – frozen or fresh
- ¼ cup mango, chopped
- 2 cups almond milk, chilled
- 14 almonds
- ½ cup oatmeal

Directions

1. Put all the ingredients into the blender and whizz up until smooth.

Almond Smoothie for the Skin

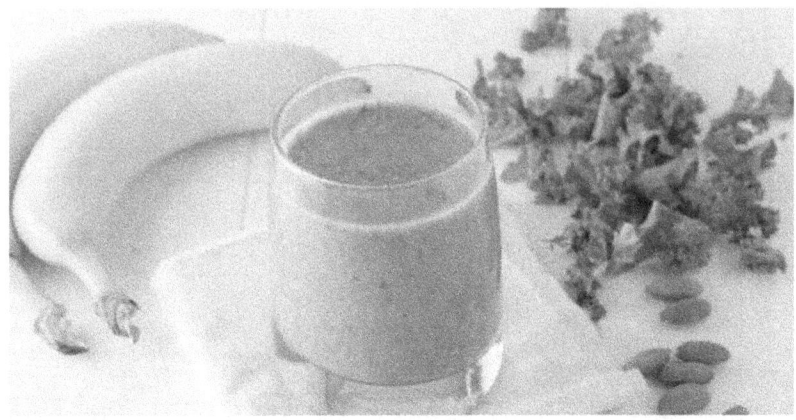

(Serves 2)

Ingredients

- 1½ cups water
- 1 cup almond milk
- 1 cup kale
- 1 cup peaches
- 1 banana
- 1 cup oats
- ¼ cup almonds

Directions

1. Put all the ingredients into the blender and whizz up until smooth.

Mango Masterpiece Smoothie

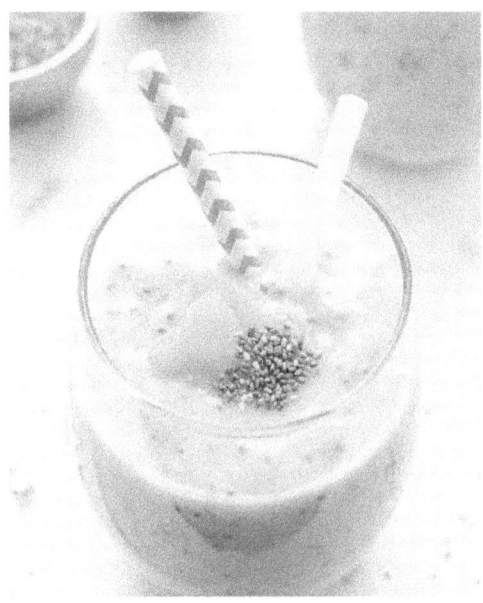

(Serves 1)

Ingredients

- 1/2 cup fresh or frozen mango
- 1 cup almond milk
- 1/2 cup clover or a leafy sprout of your choice
- 1 tablespoon Chia seeds (Cover with water and allow to soak overnight in order to thicken)
- 1 tablespoon lime juice
- 1 tablespoon stevia or honey
- 1 tablespoon almond butter
- ½ cup oatmeal

Directions

1. Put all ingredients into blender and blend until smooth. Serve over crushed ice if you want to. You should ideally always soak Chia seeds before using them.

High Protein Strawberry Smoothie

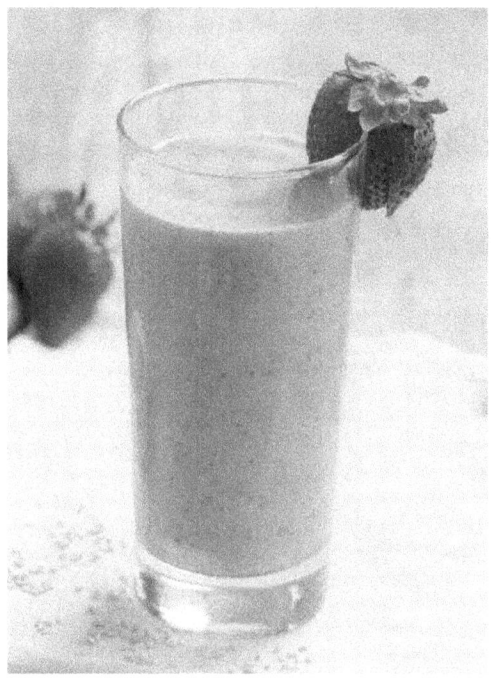

(Serves 1)

Ingredients

- 1-1/2 cups fresh strawberries, quartered
- 1/3 cup reduced fat cottage cheese
- 1/2 cup fat free milk
- 1 cup crushed ice
- 1 tsp chia seeds
- 2 to 3 fresh stevia leaves (optional)
- 1 tablespoon coconut oil
- ½ cup oat bran

Directions

1. Put all the ingredients into the blender and blend till smooth. More ice can be added to taste. Cottage cheese makes for an interesting contrast with the strawberries in this smoothie.

Belly Taming Basil Smoothie

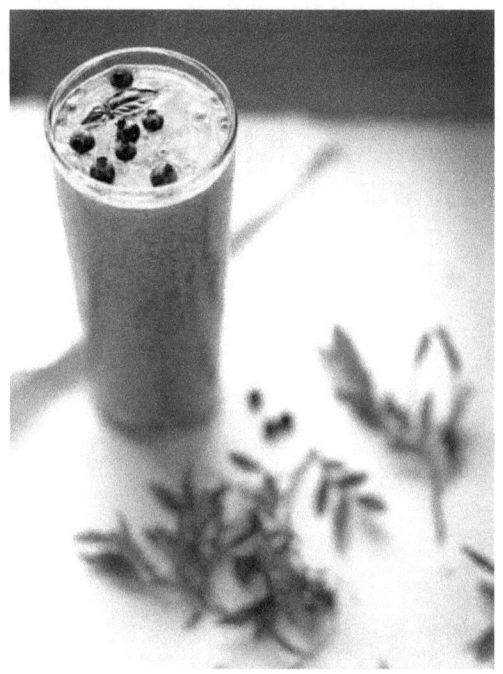

(Serves 1)

Ingredients

- 2 cups frozen blueberries
- 1 frozen banana
- ½-1 cup almond milk
- ¼ cup (5-6 leaves) fresh basil
- 3 tablespoons 2% plain Greek Yogurt
- 1 tablespoon lemon juice
- ½ avocado
- ½ cup oatmeal

Directions

1. Add all the ingredients except the almond milk. Start with half a cup of almond milk and add more if necessary. Blend well and serve immediately. This smoothie has a very distinctive flavor and is bound to become a firm favorite.

Sweet and Sour Fun

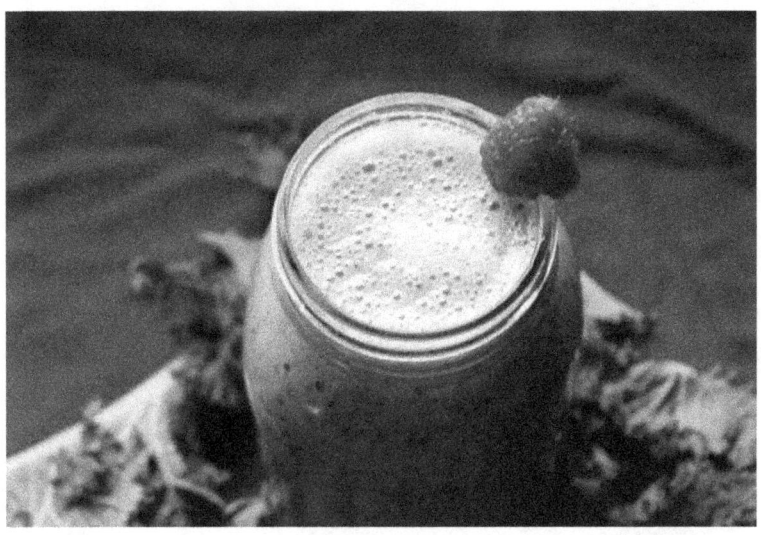

(Serves 1)

Ingredients

- 1 cup almond milk
- 1 tablespoon flaxseed, crushed just before adding
- 1 cup raspberries
- 1 banana
- ¼ cup kale
- 2 tsp lemon

Directions

1. Add all the ingredients except the almond milk. Start with half a cup of almond milk and add more if necessary. Blend well and serve immediately.

Decadence Smoothie

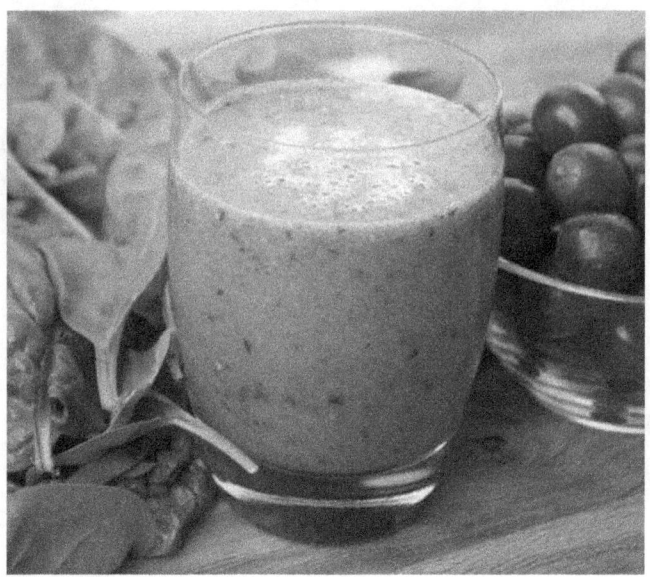

(Serves 2)

Ingredients

- 2 cups spinach, fresh
- 2 cups almond milk
- 2 cups red grapes
- 2 bananas
- 4 tablespoons almond butter

Directions

1. Whizz everything up in the blender until smooth. Serve it as is or over ice. You can swop the spinach for any other leafy green if you want to.

Cranberry Soother

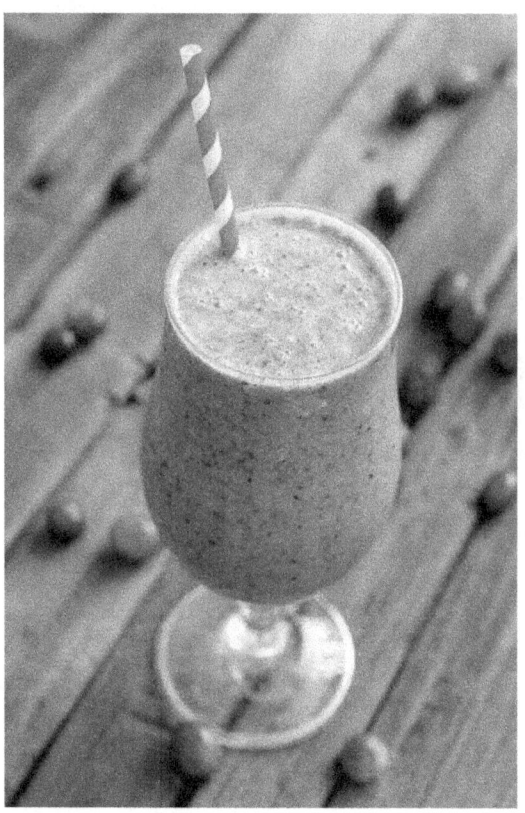

(Serves 2)

Ingredients

- 2 cups kale, fresh
- 1 cup coconut milk
- 1 cup cranberries
- 2 oranges, peeled
- 2 bananas
- 1 tablespoon coconut oil

- ¼ cup coconut flakes
- ¼ cup oatmeal

Directions

1. Whizz everything up in the blender until smooth. Serve it as is or over ice. Cranberries are really good for treating urinary tract infections so include them if you have problems in this area.

Choc-Cherry Dream Smoothie

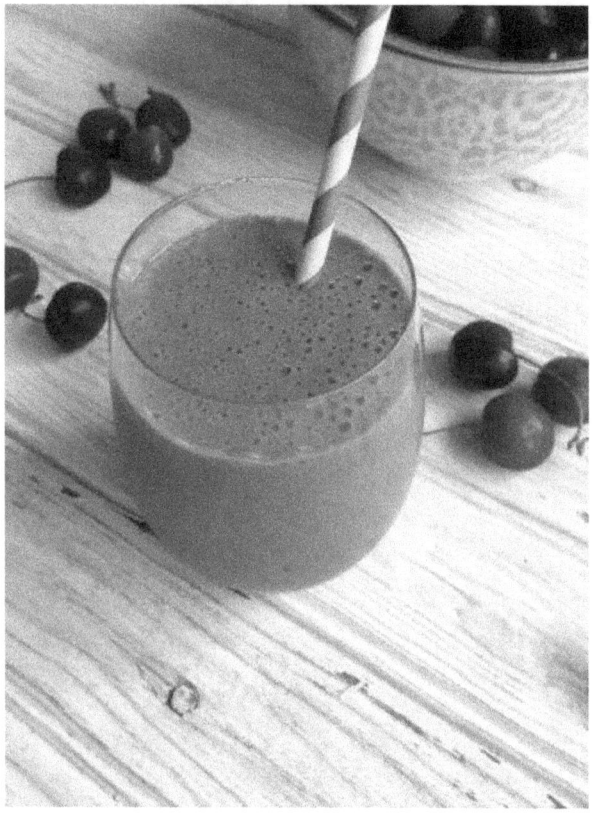

(Serves 1)

Ingredients

- ½ cup frozen cherries
- ½ cup Greek yoghurt
- ½ cup almond milk
- 1 tablespoon cocoa
- 1 teaspoon raw honey

Directions

1. Whizz everything up in the blender until smooth. Serve it as is or over ice. The combination of cocoa and honey give this smoothie a rich chocolate flavor, without all the sugar and fat of the real thing.

I hope you have learned something from this book so far and would greatly appreciate it if you could leave an honest review on Amazon.com.

Chapter Nine

Dinner Smoothies

As you will no doubt have noticed, the emphasis for smoothies during the day is to provide maximum energy possible. When it comes to dinner, we want to shift that emphasis a little.

Here we want to add ingredients that will give stabilize your blood sugar throughout the night. Did you know that sugar levels that are too high or too low can interfere with a good night's sleep?

We are also going to add in more ingredients to help relax and calm you so that you can prepare for bed.

Bananas, for example, have a lot of Magnesium in them and this is very calming, despite the amount of sugar in the fruit itself.

Lettuce is another useful item for night-time smoothies – you wouldn't think so looking at it but the humble lettuce is great for helping you get to sleep. It has calming properties and can help banish anxiety.

Here are your night-time smoothies.

Simply Soothing Smoothie

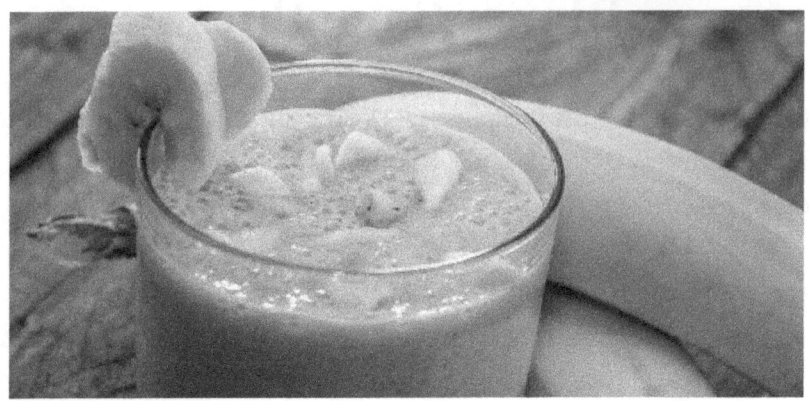

(Serves 1)

Ingredients

- 1/4 cup oats
- 1/2 cup Greek yogurt
- 1 banana, cut into thirds
- 1/2 cup almond milk
- 2 teaspoons honey
- 1/4 teaspoon cinnamon

Directions

1. Blend everything in your blender. Serve immediately.

Chocolate Berry Smoothie

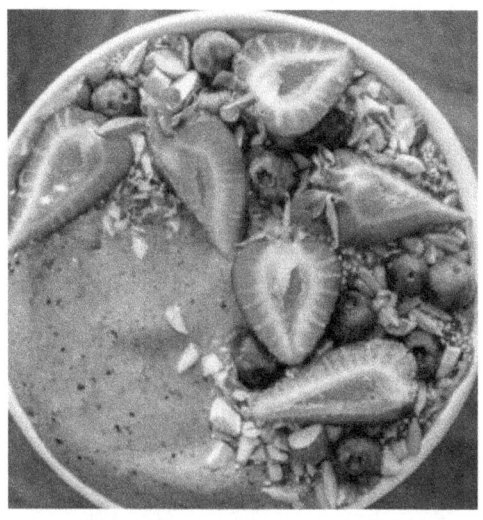

(Serves 1)

Ingredients

- 1/2 banana, peeled
- 1/2 cup blueberries
- 5 large strawberries
- 1 tablespoon cocoa powder
- 2 tablespoons chia seeds, soaked for 5 minutes
- 1 cup almond milk
- ½ cup oatmeal
- ¼ teaspoon cinnamon

Directions

1. Blend everything in your blender. Serve immediately.

Blueberry Fizz

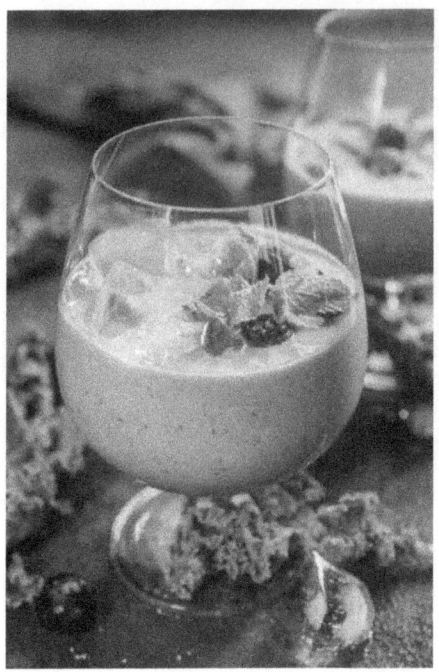

(Serves 1)

Ingredients

- ½ cup mango
- 1 cup blueberries
- 1 ½ cups coconut water/ almond milk
- 1 cup kale
- 1 tablespoon lemon juice
- ¼ avocado
- ¼ teaspoon cayenne pepper
- 1 tablespoon pumpkin seeds

Directions

1. Whizz everything up in the blender until smooth. Serve it as is or over ice. The cayenne pepper in this smoothie is not as overpowering as you might think.

Weight Loss Wonder

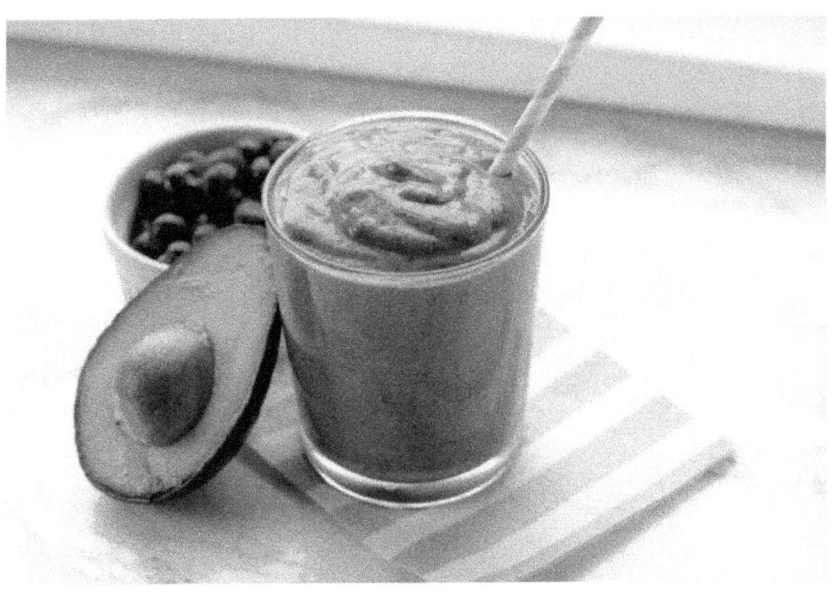

(Serves 1)

Ingredients

- 1 cup water
- 1/2 medium avocado
- 1/2 cup fresh or frozen blueberries
- 1 tablespoon chia seeds or chia seed gel
- 1/2 tablespoon coconut oil (increase to 1 tablespoon over the course of a week)
- 1/4 teaspoon cinnamon
- 1/2 tablespoon honey (optionally use stevia or maple syrup or 1/2 banana to sweeten)
- ½ cup oats

Directions

1. Whizz everything up in the blender until smooth. Serve it as is or over ice. Maple syrup will do at a push as a sweetener – just ensure that it is organic and as pure as possible.

Choc-Nut Surprise Smoothie

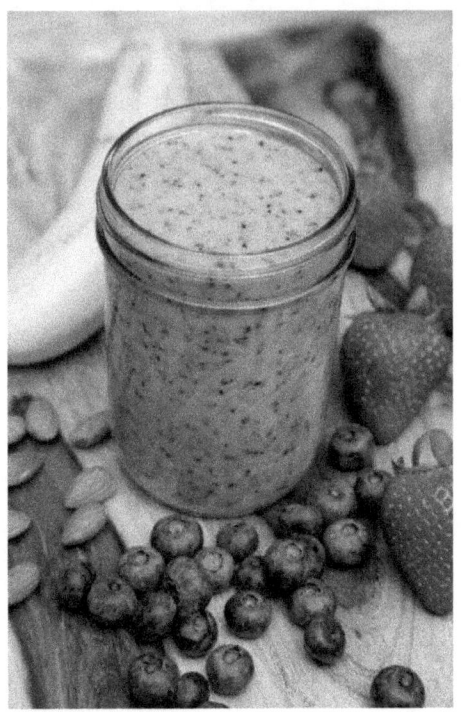

(Serves 1)

Ingredients

- 1 cup almond milk
- 1/4 cup fresh or frozen blueberries
- 1/4 cup fresh or frozen raspberries
- 1/4 cup almonds
- 1 tablespoon grass-fed butter
- 1 tablespoon cacao powder
- 1/4 teaspoon cinnamon
- 1/4 teaspoon vanilla extract

- 1/4 cup fresh or frozen strawberries
- 1/2 tablespoon cacao nibs
- 1 cup lettuce

Directions

1. Whizz everything up in the blender until smooth. Serve it as is or over ice. The cacao nibs combined with the coco powder are wonderfully rich. This smoothie is reminiscent of pudding.

Pina Colada Smoothie

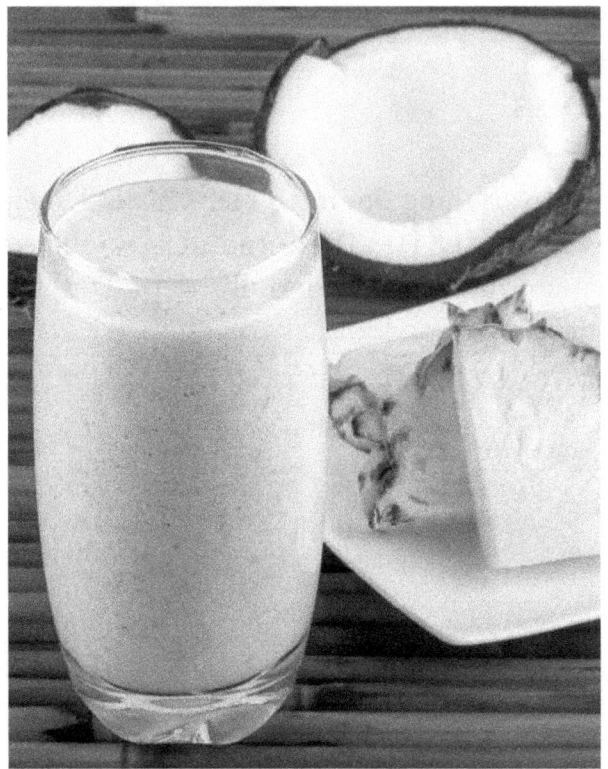

(Serves 1)

Ingredients

- 1/2 cup milk of choice
- 1 cup frozen pineapple chunks
- 1/2 cup Greek yogurt
- 1/4 teaspoon vanilla extract
- 1 teaspoon raw honey
- 3 – 5 ice cubes
- 1 tablespoon coconut flakes or shreds

- 1 teaspoon coconut oil
- 1 cup lettuce
- 1 tablespoon chia or pumpkin seeds

Directions

1. Whizz everything up in the blender until smooth. Serve it as is or over ice.

Sunset Surprise

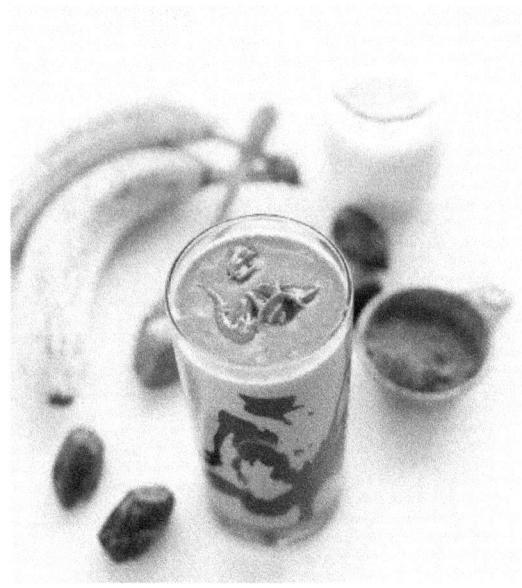

(Serves 1)

Ingredients

- 2 tbsp cocoa powder
- 2 tbsp peanut butter
- 1 banana
- 1 small tub Greek yoghurt
- ¼ teaspoon cinnamon
- ½ cup oatmeal

Directions

1. Whizz everything up in the blender until smooth. Serve it as is or over ice.

Blueberry Sundowner Smoothie

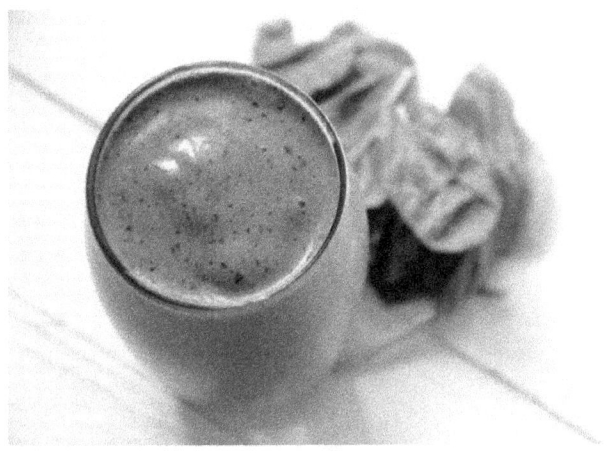

(Serves 1)

Ingredients

- 2 medium plums, pitted
- 1 cup frozen wild blueberries
- 1 head romaine lettuce
- ½ cup oatmeal
- ½ banana
- 1 cup natural yoghurt
- ½ cup water
- ¼ teaspoon cinnamon
- 1 tablespoon coconut oil

Directions

1. Whizz everything up in the blender until smooth. Serve it as is or over ice.

My Ginger Green Smoothie Recipe

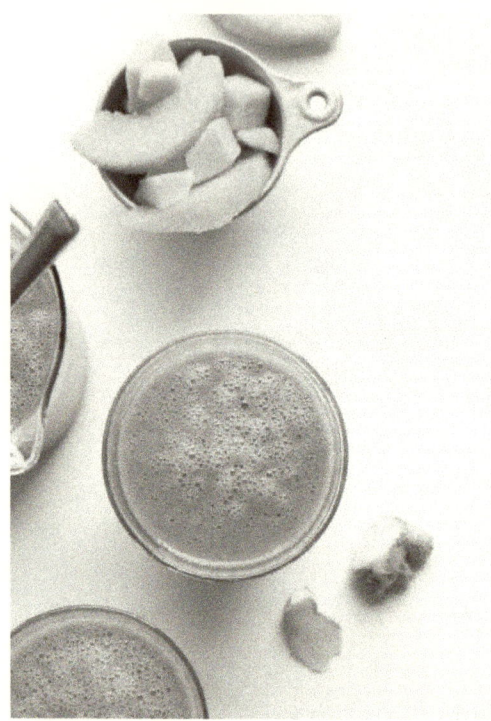

(Makes 1 large serving)

Ingredients

- 1 mango, peeled and pitted
- 2 oranges, peeled and deseeded
- 3 cups romaine lettuce, chopped
- 2 cups baby spinach
- 1/2 inch of fresh ginger root, grated or sliced
- 2 tablespoons of chia seeds, soaked for 20 minutes
- ½ cup natural yoghurt
- ½ cup water

- 1 tablespoon turmeric
- 4 or 5 corns of black pepper
- 1 teaspoon raw honey

Directions

1. Whizz everything up in the blender until smooth. Serve it as is or over ice. This sounds like lot of greens to eat at night but, as long as you don't leave eating it too late, you'll be fine.

Tummy Soother Smoothie

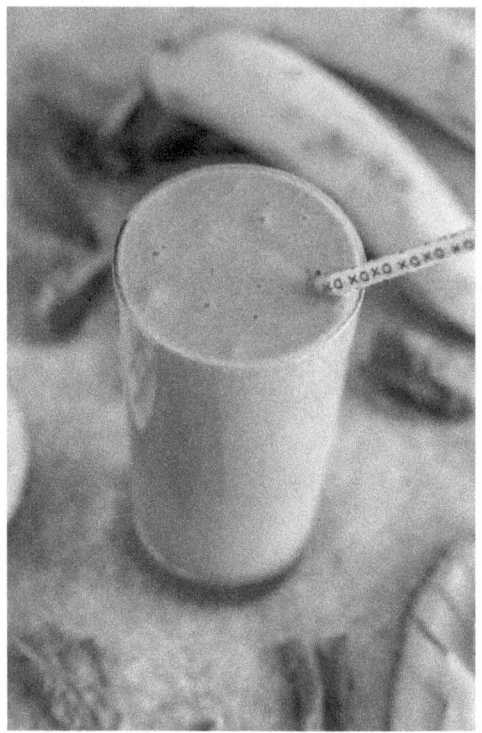

(Serves 1)

Ingredients

- 1 banana
- 1 cup kale
- 1 large sweet apple
- 1 cup chopped cucumber
- 1 stalk celery
- 1 cup lettuce
- 1/4 cup frozen mango
- 1/3 cup fresh mint leaves

- 1/2 tablespoon virgin coconut oil
- ¼ cup oatmeal

Directions

1. Whizz everything up in the blender until smooth. Serve it as is or over ice.

Chapter Ten

Mini-Smoothies

Snack smoothies do break some of the rules – you don't need to add fillers or even a lot of protein. The idea here is to provide a less calorie dense snack that you can fall back on if you find you are hungry between meals.

These smoothies will give just enough of a boost in energy and will enable you to stick to your cleanse.

Do NOT have more than two of the mini-smoothies a day. They still have calories in them, even though these are not as much as the others. It is better if you can do without the snack smoothies so do only have them if you are really not coping with the main smoothies only.

There are some smoothies in this section designed to target specific health issues.

If you find that you cannot manage a snack smoothie as well as your meal smoothies, convert the recipe of your choice to either a breakfast or lunch smoothie.

Just see what vital smoothie elements are missing and work from there.

Ice Cream Cheat Smoothie

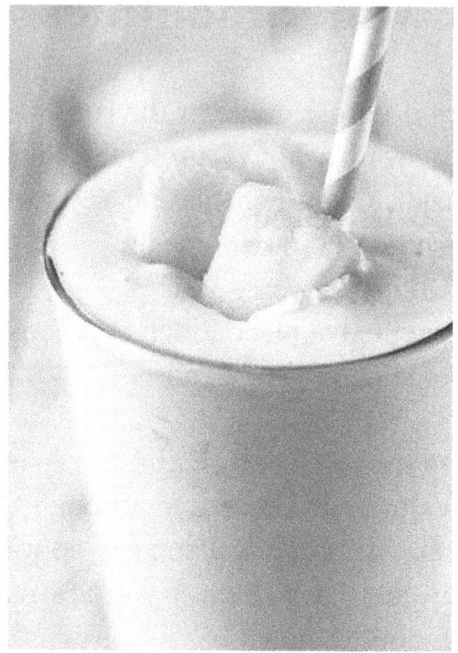

(Serves 1)

Ingredients

- 1 cup Greek yoghurt
- 1 cup pineapple
- 1 teaspoon vanilla extract
- Ice to taste

Directions

1. Whizz everything up in the blender until smooth. Serve it as is or over ice.

Ice Queen Smoothie

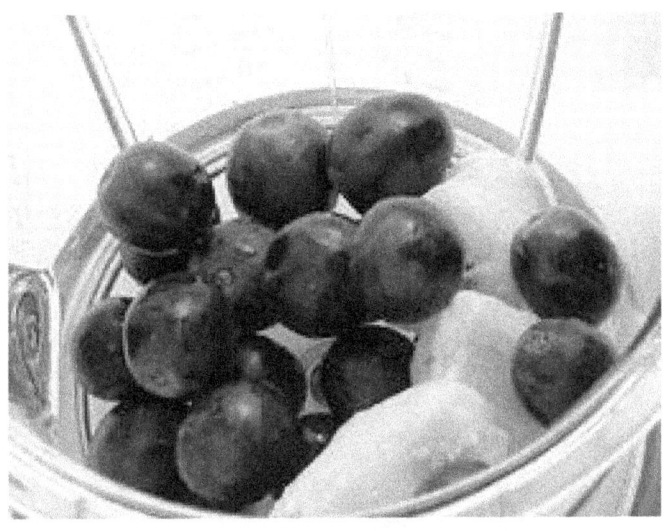

(Makes 1 large serving)

Ingredients

- 1 cup of leafy greens or sprouts of your choice
- 1 large orange, peeled or 1 large grapefruit peeled
- 1 cup coconut water
- 1/2 cup frozen grapes OR frozen watermelon
- 1/2 banana
- 1/2 cup ice

Directions

1. Whizz everything up in the blender until smooth. Add water if necessary to thin the smoothie out a little. Serve it as is, or over ice.

Blackberry Ginger Smoothie

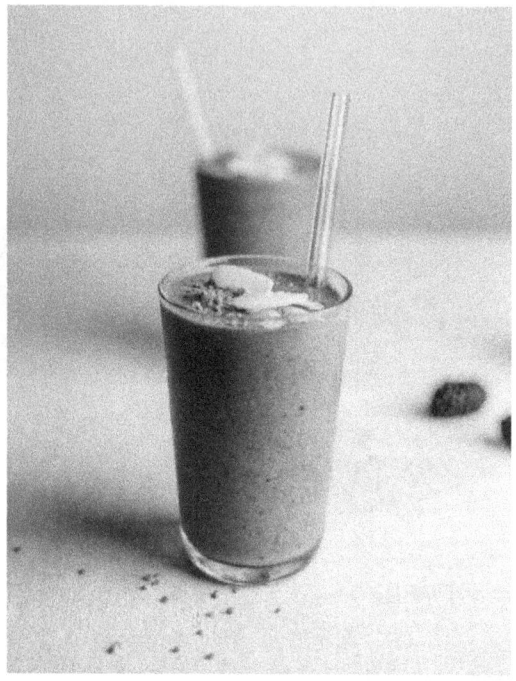

(Serves 1)

Ingredients

- 1 cup frozen blackberries
- 1 apple
- 1 banana, peeled
- 3 handfuls spinach
- 1 thumb-sized piece of fresh ginger
- ½ cup oats
- 1 cup coconut water
- 1 orange, peeled

Directions

1. Whizz everything up in the blender until smooth. Add water if necessary to thin the smoothie out a little. Serve it as is, or over ice.

Apricot Heaven

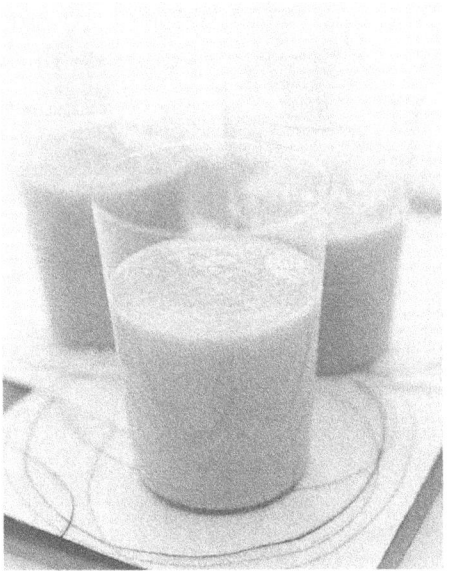

(Serves 2)

Ingredients

- 6 apricots, pitted
- 2 mangoes, pitted and peeled
- 1 cup Greek yoghurt
- 4 teaspoons fresh lemon juice
- 1 teaspoon vanilla extract
- About a cup of ice

Directions

1. Whizz everything up in the blender until smooth. Serve it as is or over ice.

Banana and Strawberry Smoothie Surprise

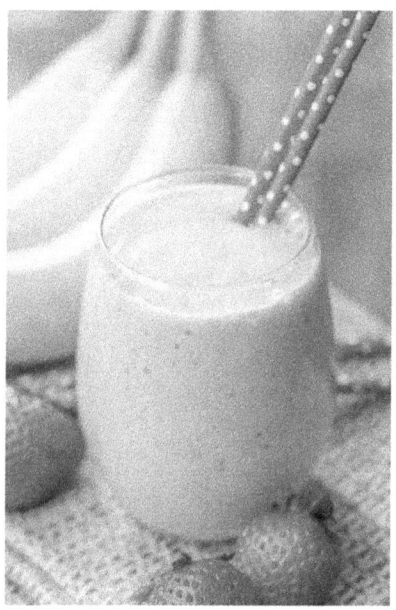

(Serves 2)

Ingredients

- 1 banana
- 1/4 cup strawberries
- 1/3 cup low fat milk
- 1 cup low fat plain yoghurt

Directions

1. Whizz everything up in the blender until smooth. Serve it as is or over ice.

Berry Dream Smoothie

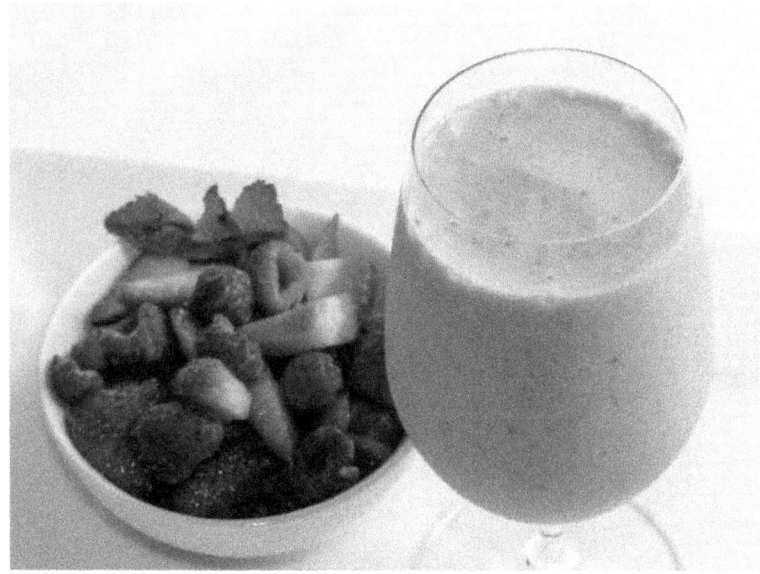

(Serves 2)

Ingredients

- 1 cup low fat raspberry yogurt
- 1/2 cup milk
- 1 cup frozen raspberries
- 3/4 cup frozen strawberries
- 2 cups of ice

Directions

1. Whizz everything up in the blender until smooth. Serve it as is or over ice.

Easy Energy Smoothie

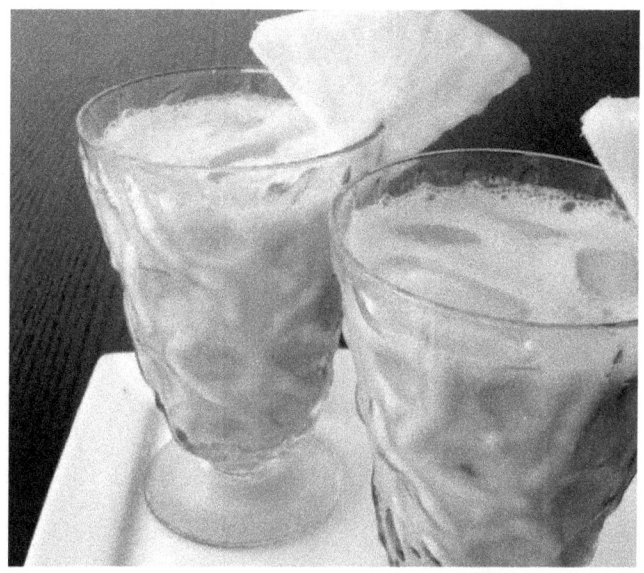

(Serves 1)

Ingredients

- ½ cup pineapple
- 1 cup watermelon
- 1 cup coconut water
- 1 cup kale
- ½ cup blueberries
- 1 green apple

Directions

1. Whizz everything up in the blender until smooth. Serve it as is or over ice.

Vitamin Boost

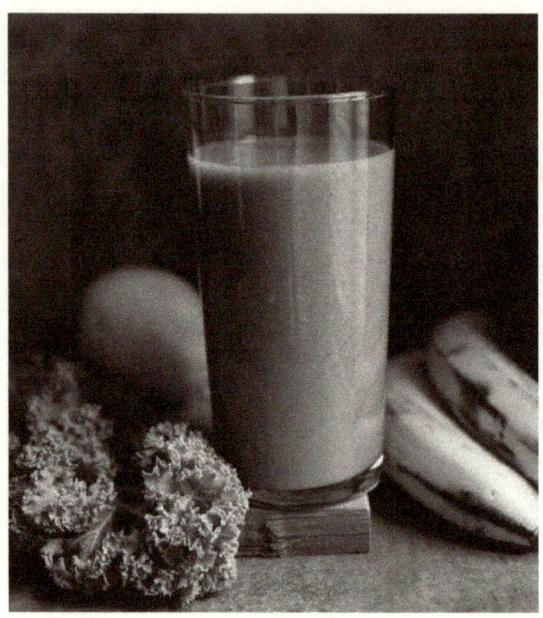

(Serves 1)

Ingredients

- 1 cup papaya
- 1/2 cup kale
- 1/2 cup spinach
- 1/2 banana
- 1/2 green apple

Directions

1. Whizz everything up in the blender until smooth. Serve it as is or over ice.

Purely Refreshing Smoothie

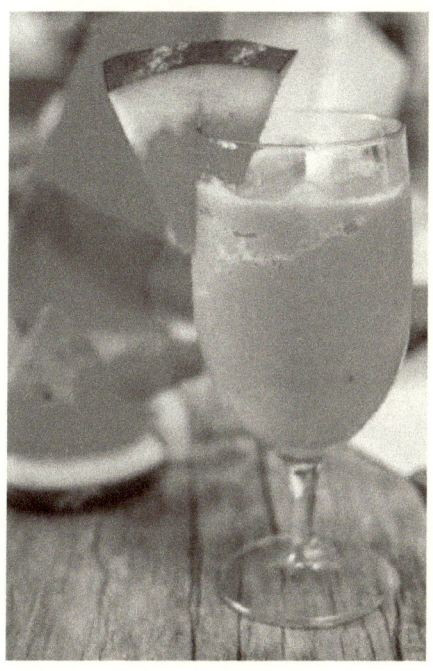

(Serves 2)

Ingredients

- 2 cups watermelon
- ¼ cup milk
- 2 cups ice

Directions

1. Whizz everything up in the blender until smooth. Serve it immediately for a refreshing cooler on a hot summer's day.

Cold and Flu Fighter

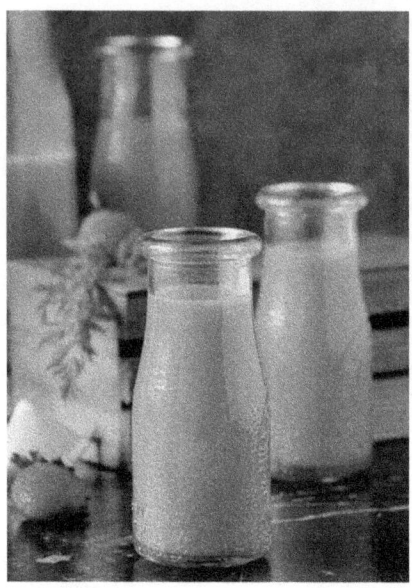

(Serves 1)

Ingredients

- 2 oranges (peeled)
- 1 cup melon
- 1 cup strawberries
- 1 tomato

Directions

1. Whizz everything up in the blender until smooth. Serve it as is or over ice. This is the first of the "medicinal" smoothies and should be drunk at the first sign of a cold or flu.

Go Go Goji Berries

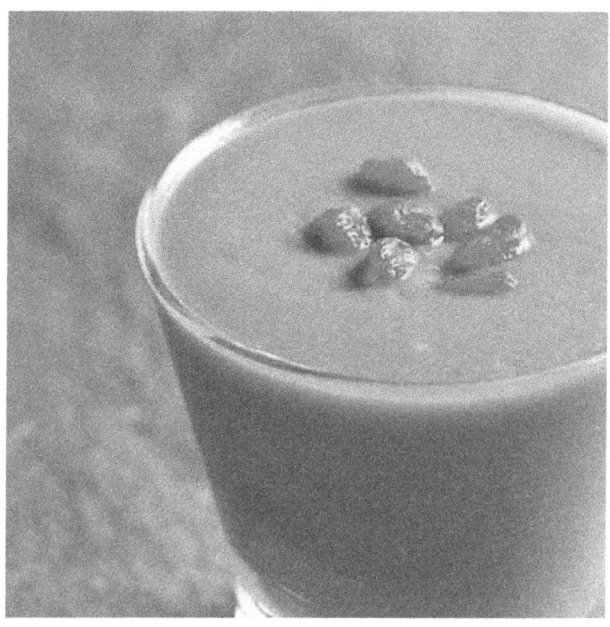

(Serves 2)

Ingredients

- 4 stalks of celery, chopped
- 1bananas, fresh or frozen
- 1/2 cup Goji berries, soaked in water for 20 minutes
- 1 cup mango pieces, fresh or frozen
- 1 cup coconut water

Directions

1. Whizz everything up in the blender until smooth. Serve it as is or over ice.

Peaches and Dream Smoothie

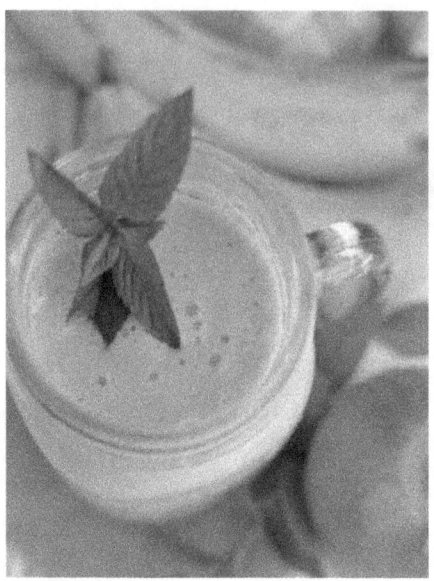

(Makes 1 Large Serving)

Ingredients

- 1 peach, pitted
- 1 banana
- 1 small bunch grapes
- 1 carrot
- ¼ cup oatmeal
- 1 cup milk

Directions

1. Whizz everything up in the blender until smooth. Serve it as is or over ice.

Berry Berry Citrus Smoothie

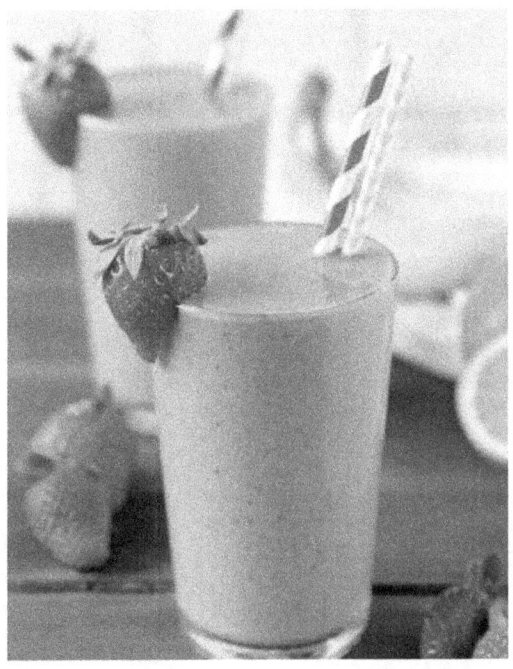

(Serves 1)

Ingredients

- 1/2 banana, cut in chunks, frozen
- ½ cup strawberries, frozen
- 1 orange, peeled
- 1/2 cup almond milk

Directions

1. Whizz everything up in the blender until smooth. Serve it as is or over ice.

Smoothie to Treat Gout

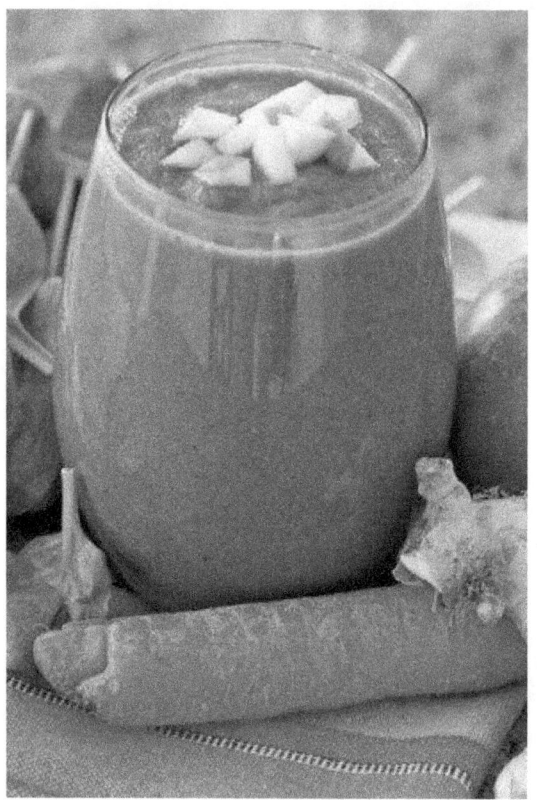

(Serves 2)

Ingredients

- 2 green apples
- 2 carrots
- 2 cups kale
- Juice of half a lemon
- 1 piece of ginger as big as your thumb

Directions

1. Whizz everything up in the blender until smooth. Serve it as is or over ice. You will find that the smoothie cleanse will go a long way to clearing up the gout on its own. After the cleanse, drink one of these a day and gout will become a distant memory.

Smoothie to Boost Anti-Oxidants

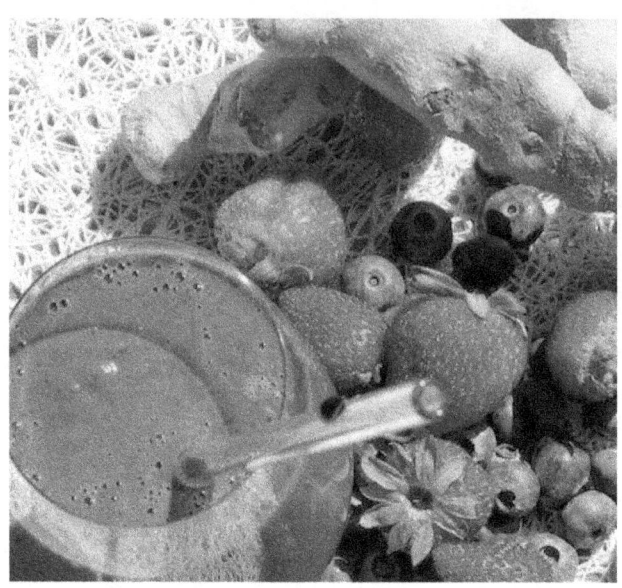

Ingredients

- 3 tablespoons hemp powder
- A thumb-sized piece of ginger
- 2 cups of leafy greens or sprouts
- 1 stalk celery
- 1 cup of frozen berries
- ½ to 1 cup cooled green tea

Directions

1. Whizz everything up in the blender until smooth. Serve it as is or over ice. The green tea is a superb anti-oxidant and actually boosts your body's ability to take up and use more anti-oxidants.

Smoothie to Beat Inflammation

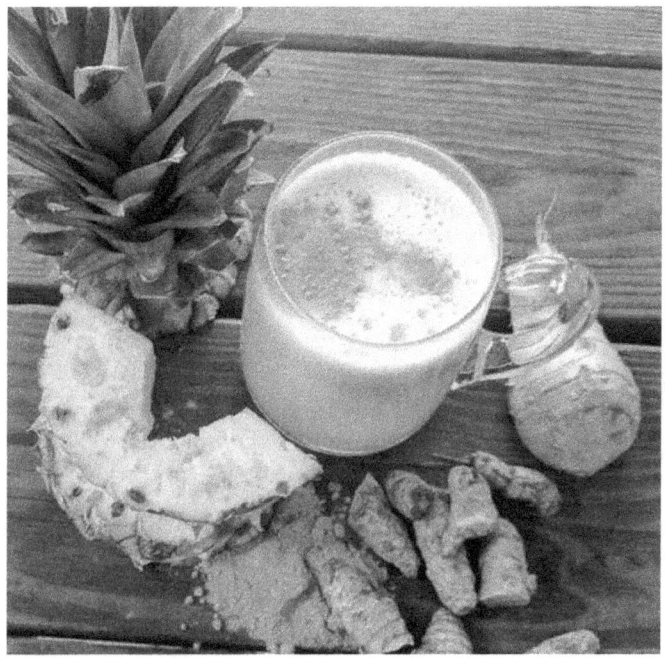

(Serves 1)

Ingredients

- 1 cup coconut water
- 1 cup water, coconut water or cold green tea
- 1 cup pineapple
- 2 tablespoons turmeric
- 1 thumb-sized piece of ginger
- 1 teaspoon chia or flaxseeds
- Handful of macadamia nuts
- 1/2 cup ice

Directions

1. Whizz everything up in the blender until smooth. Serve it as is or over ice. If you suffer with chronic inflammatory disease like rheumatism or arthritis, one of these smoothies daily will go a long way to improving your quality of life.

Smoothie for an Upset Stomach

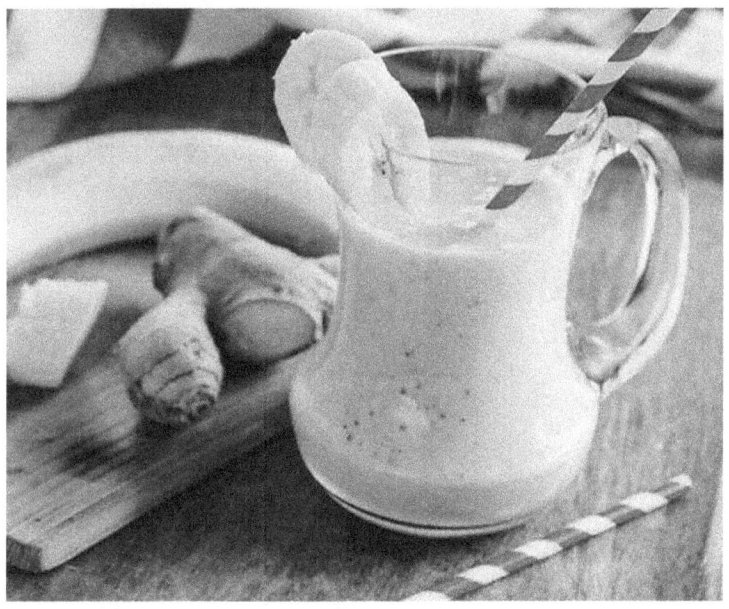

(Serves 2)

Ingredients

- 1 banana
- ¾ Greek yoghurt
- 1 tablespoon honey
- 1 teaspoon vanilla extract
- ½ teaspoon fresh grated ginger

Directions

1. Whizz everything up in the blender until smooth. Serve it as is or over ice.

Triple-Punch Antioxidant Boost

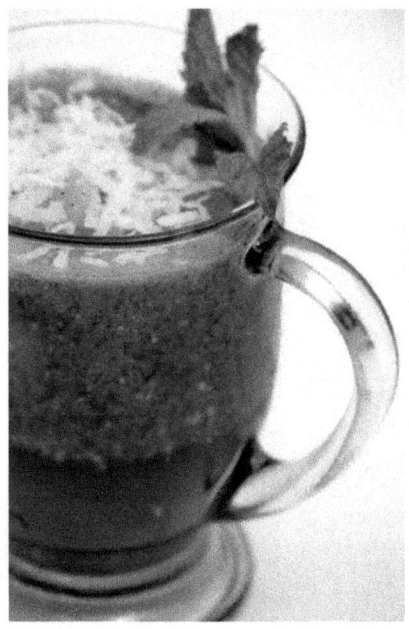

(Serves 1)

Ingredients

- ¾ cup coconut milk
- ¼ cup boiling water
- 1 teabag of green tea
- 2 teaspoons
- Honey
- 1 ½ cup blueberries – fresh or frozen
- 1 medium carrot
- ½ banana
- ½ cup wheat grass

Directions

1. Allow the teabag to soak in the water and leave to cool. Add the water and other ingredients to the blender. Whizz everything up in the blender until smooth. Serve it as is or over ice.

Don't forget to share your thoughts on this book by leaving a review on Amazon.com. It takes just a few seconds.

Discover Scientifically-Proven "Shortcuts" & "Hacks" to Lose Weight FASTER (With Very Little Effort)

For this month only, you can get Linda's best-selling & most popular book absolutely free – *Weight Loss Secrets You NEED to Know.*

Get Your FREE Copy Here:
TopFitnessAdvice.com/Bonus

Discover scientifically-proven tips to help you lose weight faster and easier than ever before. With this book, readers were able to improve their weight loss results and fitness levels. So, it's highly recommended that you get this book, especially while it's free!

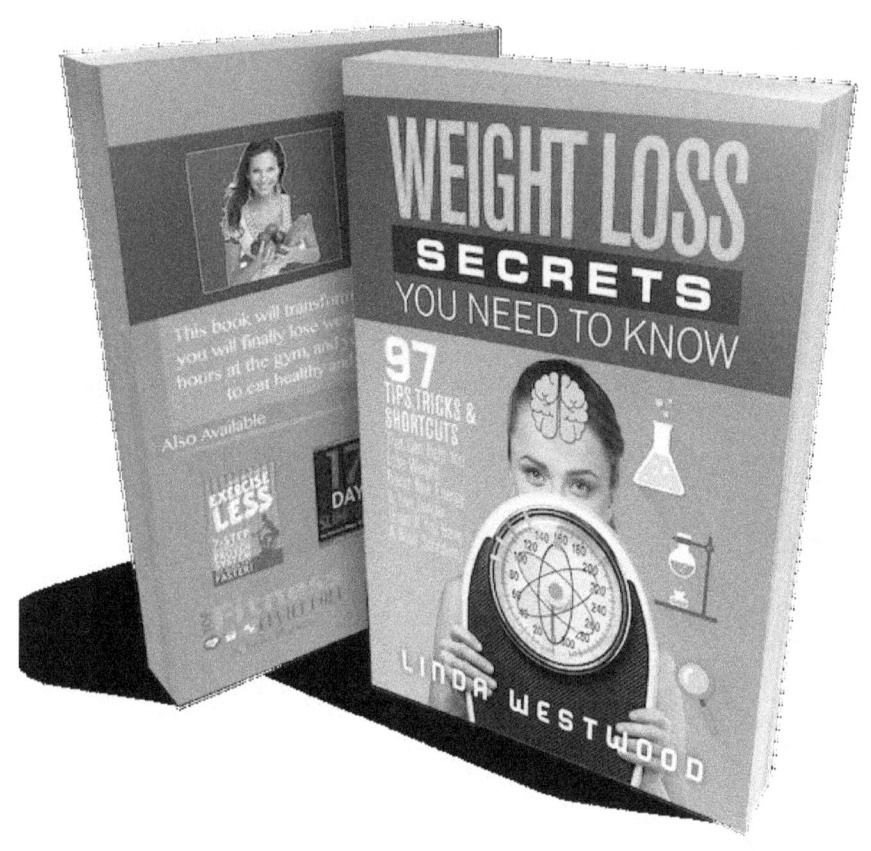

Get Your FREE Copy Here:
TopFitnessAdvice.com/Bonus

Conclusion

So, there you have it – the 9-Day Smoothie Cleanse.

As you can see, the reason that this plan is so effective is that you are given a lot of freedom – it does not feel as though you are on diet at all. Your green tea allows you to get some caffeine to take the edge off but also boosts your body's fat-burning centers.

You do not feel deprived because there is plenty to "eat" and the smoothies taste great. The smoothies contain enough nutrients to ensure that you have loads of energy to tackle the day and enough fiber to ensure that you never feel hungry.

You end by losing weight and feeling like you have the energy to take on the whole world. You'll never want to stop once you get into it. I encourage you to play around and find smoothie recipes that you love.

Good luck and all the best for your slimmer future!

Enjoying this book?

Check out my other best sellers!

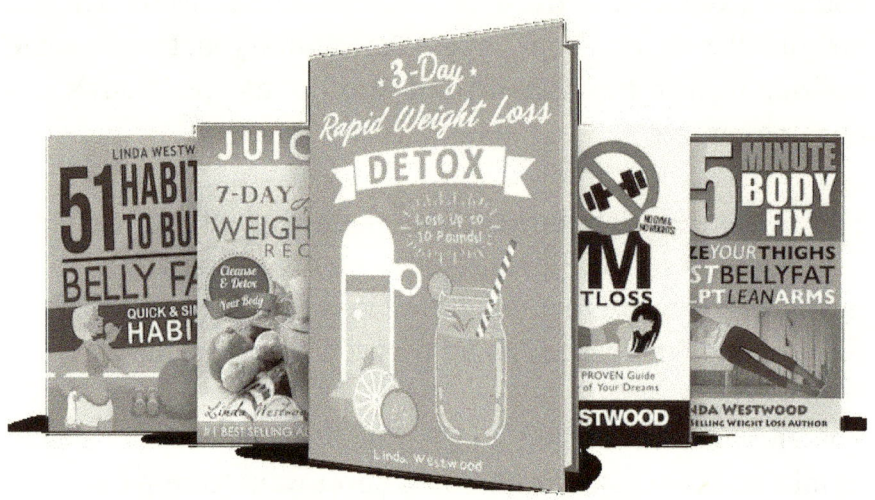

Get your next book on sale here:

TopFitnessAdvice.com/go/books

Final Words

I would like to thank you for purchasing my book and I hope I have been able to help you and educate you on something new.

If you have enjoyed this book and would like to share your positive thoughts, could you please take 30 seconds of your time to go back and give me a review on my Amazon book page.

I greatly appreciate seeing these reviews because it helps me share my hard work.

You can leave me a review on Amazon.com.

Again, thank you and I wish you all the best!

www.ingramcontent.com/pod-product-compliance
Lightning Source LLC
Chambersburg PA
CBHW031152020426
42333CB00013B/630